Don't Eat the Elephants

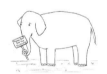

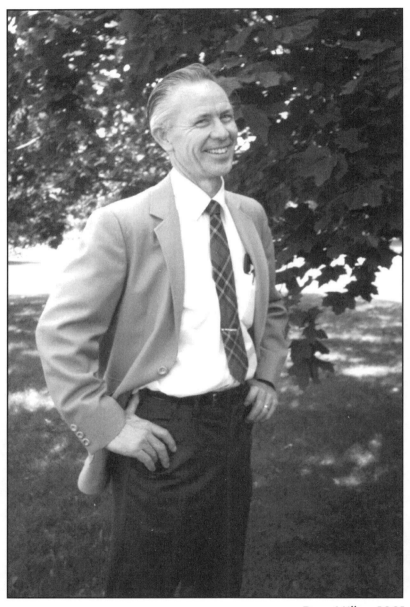

Don Miller, 1981

Don't Eat the Elephants

by Patricia H. Miller
edited by Diana E. Brown

Pocahontas Press, Inc.
Blacksburg, Virginia

Don't Eat the Elephants, by Patricia H. Miller
Diana E. Brown, editor
Cover design by Sarah Kamppila, Virginia Tech,
Blacksburg, Virginia

Published by Pocahontas Press, Inc., Blacksburg, VA 24063
Printed in the United States of America by
McNaughton & Gunn, Inc., Saline, Michigan 48176

ISBN 0-936015-98-5
First printing 2006

This book is written for,
and dedicated to,
Don Miller,
with all my love.

It is also dedicated
with heartfelt thanks to all
who walked pieces of this road with our family,
and helped make the load a little lighter,
and the road a little brighter.

And, dedicated with much respect to
all who have walked,
all who are walking,
and those who assist others
who make their way down a similar path.

This is a true story. I am sharing our experiences with the hope that they may be of some help to others who face similar challenges.

To protect privacy and anonymity, many names and places have been changed. All facilities and corporations have fictitious names or are unnamed, and any similarity to any existing facility or corporation is coincidental and unintentional.

Acknowledgments

First of all, my thanks to my long-time friend, Diana Brown of New Markets, Unlimited, Atlanta, Georgia. Without the support, encouragement, guidance, editing, and expertise of all kinds that she provided, I'm not at all sure this story would be in book form.

In an effort to keep my emotional balance during the years that Don was ill, I recorded events, and poured my thoughts and feelings onto paper. After his death, I found myself with 14 steno books and numerous typewritten pages crammed full of notes and documented information. It was Diana who encouraged me to type those notes into my computer, suggesting that I not worry about organizing or formatting. Later, she helped me arrange the material into story form and acceptable format, and edited what I wrote. Her "Show, don't tell!" was only one of the repeated suggestions that began to ring in my ears as I sought to understand and utilize the many writing skills she shared.

I gratefully acknowledge the profession of Occupational Therapy, which teaches and validates the importance of seeing the person, and not the disease, in order to provide compassionate and quality care.

My thanks to all the friends who took the time to read my manuscript-in-progress and offer their inputs and encouragement.

And my thanks to Mary Holliman and Pocahontas Press for taking this project on and patiently guiding me through the process of getting our story published.

Chapter One

A young woman ushered us into a small room, and left.

Don perched awkwardly on the examining table. I sat down on the little chair beside it.

And we waited.

Finally, the doctor walked in. He looked directly at me, almost ignoring Don, and after a few preliminaries brusquely declared, "Your husband has Alzheimer's disease."

Speechless, I simply stared at the man for a few moments.

"Could it possibly be depression?" I asked when I found my voice.

"He's not depressed, and you are in denial," was his cold response.

Denial? I hadn't had time to accept or deny anything. But this diagnosis couldn't possibly be right. My handsome, fit, barely 59-year-old husband could not have Alzheimer's. No way.

I was appalled and stunned by the doctor's unbelievable declarations, and angered by the way the words were delivered. I struggled to keep those emotions and my building panic in check, as we briefly discussed the situation. Then, with no desire to communicate further with this less than compassionate doctor, I said, "goodbye." My hand reached for Don's as instinctively as his reached for mine, and we walked out of that man's office, down the steps, and toward our car.

As we walked in silence across the parking lot on that sunny October afternoon in 1988, neither one of us was basking in the beauty of the colorful fall leaves that surrounded us. Don was evidently processing what we had just heard, and when we arrived at the car his words suddenly erupted.

"I'll head for the river first!"

That river was less than a mile from our home . . . and his vow struck even more fear into my heart. But I identified with his outburst! How would I react to hearing such a diagnosis, such a cruel pronouncement of my own death sentence?

I didn't know how to respond. Then I remembered the picture Don had slipped across the dinner table long ago, and the words rolled out. "No elephants, Don. We mustn't 'eat elephants' — we've got to take just one step at a time. This doctor doesn't know for sure what's wrong. There are other doctors out there we can see. And no matter what's going on, we'll walk this road together as we always have."

Don didn't respond, but he did seem to relax a bit. How I hoped he would be able to remember his simple sketch of an elephant clutching a sign that read, "Please Don't Eat the Elephants!" He had drawn it for me in the early years of our marriage, after patiently listening to my futile attempts to solve some dilemma that seemed to be overwhelming me. The more I discussed all the aspects of the situation, the more I worried about all that might happen, the bigger the whole problem seemed to become.

Over the years, we had often joked about his clever reminder, and I was always the one who needed to work the hardest at putting the concept into practice. Whether or not Don could recall the picture or its meaning on that life-changing afternoon, I knew that now it was more important than ever that I remember. How I responded to this challenge would make all the difference for both of us. And I realized almost immediately that how I responded would be the only control I would have over our situation.

Chapter Two

If I were going to start at the beginning, where would I start? Perhaps in June 1949, when I graduated from high school . . . In some ways that seems like yesterday. But in other ways it seems like a million years ago, almost like another lifetime.

That summer I worked as a secretary in San Francisco, traveling in and out of the city by commuter train from my parents' home on the Bay Area Peninsula. I was physically there, in California, yet like most teenagers, I was ready to depart, move on, be on my own.

There had been no question. College was supposed to be the next step in the plan — the often unspoken but generally understood "Plan" according to many families living in San Francisco suburbs in the 1940s — for men to obtain a degree that would enable them to support their families, and for women to obtain their "Mrs." degree. But money was not in abundant supply at our house. I had to choose. I could go to nearby Stanford and live at home, or I could attend college at the University of Idaho. I was well aware of my parents' logic. My older brother was a junior at U of I; if I chose the University of Idaho, he could keep an eye on me.

At 17 I had no problem making that choice. No living at home for me. I headed north!

One of my very first lessons involved the pronunciation of the name of this small college town nestled in the foothills of northern Idaho. In no uncertain terms, I was informed that

Moscow rhymed with low, snow, any similar word, but definitely not with cow!

That first year was filled with challenges, opportunities, fun times — all kinds of new and exciting experiences. Many extra-curricular on-campus activities centered around exchanges, dances, dates of all kinds. I began to sense a deep longing. Was there, somewhere, a special guy just for me? I began to wonder.

But even while one is thinking he or she may never appear, one never knows how or when one may meet that special person.

Late one Friday morning that spring, I was walking down "Hello Walk," a steep, picturesque path that led from the administration building and various classrooms to many student living quarters on campus. All winter long it had been a snowy, slippery, windy, and cold trip up and down that hill. But on that day I was enjoying the sun, the mild temperature, the

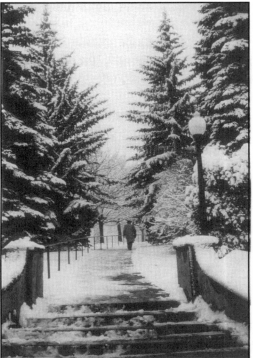

sights and smells of new growth, the jubilant atmosphere of students celebrating and enjoying the glorious weather.

I was through with classes for the day. Through with classes for the week! But for me, weekends often held an air of being not quite complete. Something, someone, that "special" someone, was missing.

As I walked down the hill that

morning, along came a good-looking young man in an "I" jacket — the maroon and white wool and leather jacket worn by many U of I athletes. This young athlete's jacket was embellished with the usual "I" for Idaho, and was also covered with a large assortment of small pins, obviously for awards in other sports.

I noticed the jacket, the pins, but what caught my attention most of all was the warm "hello" and the handsome face that carried a wonderfully engaging grin. I had seen him before. Where? Oh, yes. His name was Don Miller, and he too, was a member of the swimming club.

I was suddenly very aware of the swimming cap on top of my head. Everyone accepted into the swim club that spring was required to wear a cap all week, and I had carefully pinned mine onto my long hair with bobby pins. I had worn it each day with a mixture of self-consciousness and pride.

As I continued my way on down the hill, the self-consciousness disappeared, the pride remained, and was now mixed with a warm glow from Don's cheerful greeting. Something unique had happened in that instant of the brief look we exchanged. We had connected in a manner reminiscent of *deja vu* — connected in a way that I couldn't explain to myself . . .

My special someone had appeared.

But at that moment, I only felt the glow. I had no way of knowing intellectually what a significant and special person that young man would become in my life. Only my feelings recorded that something momentous had occurred. My walk suddenly had a spring to it, and the smile that spread across my face was a broad one. I often saw him again on campus, at swim club meetings, read his name in the paper, but it took that quiet engineering student quite a while to gather the courage to pick up the telephone and call me. Our first date was the next spring — almost a year later. It was worth waiting for.

What excitement that original phone call produced! I could hardly contain myself as I jubilantly bounced down the hall from the phone booth to share with my roommate. "That call was from Don Miller! He asked me to go to a formal dance next Friday night!" How glad I was that I already had a pretty white lace strapless formal a friend had made for me — a dress just waiting for some special occasion. The glow was back! I could hardly wait for the night of the dance to arrive.

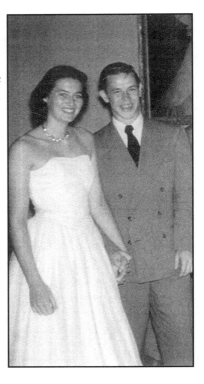

That Friday evening was like something out of a story-book for me. I found myself holding hands, dancing, laughing, sharing thoughts with Don, being his special date. It was an evening I will never forget. And in spite of the late hour that we parted that night — the night before a big track meet — Don ran a personal best and won the 440 yard dash the next afternoon, as I stood by the side of that old cinder track excitedly cheering him on.

What a delightful spring those next months became. Don and I spent many wonderful evenings together, enjoyed marvelous adventures of all kinds, then all of a sudden it was June. With it came the first of many separations. The train whisked me back to California. I would be working in San Francisco again, while Don headed for a summer job at Hayden Lake, near Coeur d' Alene, Idaho.

But two weeks later, he arrived at the University of California Berkeley campus to run in a Big Ten track meet. A glorious weekend! And, another difficult "goodbye." Our eyes, along with our hearts, were riveted on September, when we would be together again.

We kept the U.S. Postal Service busy. When I arrived home after work each evening, checking for mail was definitely the first order of business. One evening in August, enclosed within a thick envelope, I found the story of that first spring expressed in unique and heart-warming words. That fine athlete was also a poet.

'Twas during the second semester
  Of the school year '49 and '50,
I saw a girl one morning
  Who I thought was mighty nifty.

A swimming cap perched atop her head
  Made a sight I'll call amazing;
A cheery "hello" surprised me,
  Then my eyes they went appraising.

They much approved of what they saw,
  My head was in a whirl;
Could it be that I might meet
  This most attractive girl?

I started out to look for her,
  To find out her house and name;
But a full year had elapsed
  Before my big break came.

"A dance the night before a meet?"
  Stan said, "You'd best stay home, you nut."
But I've been doing that for three years now,
  I'm getting in a rut.

So I called and met with much success,
  Almost too good to be true.
But true it was, and so I had
  My first dance date with you.

I enjoyed the dance that evening,
    Like I never had before;
Went home that night determined
    To call you up some more.

So the next few months it seemed we toured
    Most everything in reach,
From the sidewalks of east Moscow
    To cold Chatcolet's rocky beach.

Yet to have a real fine evening,
    We didn't need to travel,
For I much enjoyed the times we'd sit
    And let the tales unravel.

This sort of thing was new to me,
    At times I'd really fear
That this was much too good to happen
    To a mossy engineer.

Then came the time to say "goodbye,"
    I'd not looked forward to the day,
When all too soon you'd vanish
    Down California way.

But we met again in Berkeley,
    After two weeks had gone by.
Though beaten racing, I was still all smiles,
    Chuck and Dewey, they knew why.

Spent a most enjoyable weekend there;
    Sure didn't want to go,
Cause I knew the next two months
    Would stretch out awfully slow.

So now you see how you affect me,
But I'm raising no complaint,
Except for now when things are such
That where you are . . . I ain't . . .

But I'm sure time will correct this,
Won't take but a week or two,
To be in Moscow to start
The year of '51 and '52.

But now there's an occasion
For which all this is written,
Yet I'm having trouble saying
Something that's befittin'.

I guess that I'll fall back and use
That fine, old time-worn line
Which, if I could say in person
Great pleasure would be mine.

Since I'll not be there to say it,
I'll write it down for you,
And I'll know you'll understand
That I really mean it, too.

A Happy Birthday to you, Pat,
I wish you many, many more,
And may Lady Luck present you
With good fortunes by the score.

Don

That first long summer finally came to an end. I arrived
back on campus with a huge grin on my face, a new light in my
eyes, and "wings on my heels." There was a special guy who
really cared about me. Not only someone special, but a young
man who had completely captured my heart and soul. He was

there. On campus! And so was I. The year ahead was filled with promise.

It was my junior year at the university, and Don's senior year. Amidst the demands of the full load of classes that we both carried, and the variety of outside activities in which we each participated, we still managed to find plenty of time to be together. Our relationship blossomed. We spent many hours sharing thoughts about every conceivable subject. We discovered that silence was equally comfortable. Hand in hand, we roamed the sidewalks of our campus and the little college town. We danced to the tunes of the big bands of the forties and fifties.

And, we fell in love.

Sorority house rules at the University of Idaho in the early 1950s required that young women be home, in the house, by 10:30 p.m. on week nights, and 1:00 a.m. on weekends. Each night our housemother diligently blinked the porch light five minutes before the door was closed and securely locked. Anyone not in on time was in trouble! The porch was always lined with parting couples stealing a last kiss.

In May of 1952, Don and I spent part of one pleasant Friday evening with two other couples. All of us agreed we didn't want to say goodnight at the final blink of that porch light. We didn't want the 1:00 a.m. kiss to be the last — we wanted more time together. The six of us laid careful plans. We would meet at Don's 1940 black Ford on the side road near the sorority house at 2:00 a.m. The guys would bring blankets and sleeping bags, buy food, soft drinks, and beer. We would all spend the rest of the night at nearby Lake Chatcolet.

When activity in the house settled down, the three of us cautiously headed for the sleeping porch, tiptoed past the long rows of bunk beds, quietly slipped out the third floor fire escape door and down the metal stairs. Doing our best to contain nervous laughter, we scurried across the lawn to the darkened car where the three guys waited with the motor quietly idling, all of us wondering if we would truly make it out the door and past our housemother's listening ear.

We piled into the car, and amidst giggles and hushed whispers, Don eased the car away from the curb. We were off!

At the lake we arranged blankets and sleeping bags, pulled out snacks and cold drinks, built a small fire, and gathered around it in a cozy circle to celebrate our freedom. But it wasn't long before the coals died down, before our excitement led to fatigue, and each couple found warmth curled up next to one another beneath blankets and sleeping bags.

I snuggled up next to Don, tried to get comfortable on the hard ground, then grinned as I heard Kathy's voice a few feet away.

"Bill! You're too close!"

How "good" we all were, how obedient to the mores, the accepted codes of behavior for our times. But we had snuck out of the house! And the intrigue of stepping out of line added to our sense of adventure and pleasure that lovely spring evening.

Of course, the next morning we had to get back in without raising suspicions. I had an exam at 8:00 a.m. in my Saturday shorthand class. It required no cramming, no special concern, but I did need to show up. Bright and early we all piled back into the Ford, and Don headed the car down the winding road back to town. The couples parted, and the three of us women attempted to unobtrusively walk back into the house. When I entered the large room that I shared with several others, I was greeted with a quizzical look by a younger roommate.

"If I didn't know you, I'd think you'd been on a sneak date . . ."

If she didn't know me? It is easy to look back at those early years and wonder who I truly was. I was so carefully toeing the line, following the rules, the guidelines my parents and society laid down, that I don't think I knew much about who I really was myself. But yes, I did go on a sneak date, broke all the rules to snuggle (and snuggle only) with Don Miller. And what a wonderful feeling it was to know that there was someone I cared that much about, someone with whom I even wanted to take such an exciting risk.

Several days later, I received a cartoon in the mail.

The drawing showed a professor glaring over the podium at a disheveled-looking student arriving for an exam in pajamas, with toothbrush and toothpaste in hand. "Well, Harris, glad to see you could make it," said the caption, with my maiden name actually printed there in black and white.

"This was boldly stolen from an old *Argonaut* [our U of I newspaper]," said Don's neat printing. "Thought you might get the point!"

After dancing away another lovely evening that spring, we parked on a hill overlooking the campus. The lights from the campus and nearby town twinkled below, but we were not admiring the view. Our kiss was long and passionate, and the glow that always seemed to accompany Don's presence filled my being. The mellow strains of "our" song, "Blue Moon," began to drift from the car radio, adding an extra thrill.

Then through the darkness came a quiet, "Could you put up with me on a long-term basis?"

"Oh, yes," I whispered back.

I knew what he meant. And I was certain.

Soon the inevitable June arrived, with another parting imminent. This time it was not only for the summer. Don would start his engineering career with a large corporation, work for three months, and then begin Air Force basic training in Texas the last week of August.

I would go back to the San Francisco Bay Area, live with my parents, work in the city for the summer, and return to Moscow for my last year of classes. Alone. Surrounded by people. But nevertheless, I knew I would feel very much alone.

September rolled around and I arrived back on campus, struggling to find my smile and my light-hearted step. The shiny ring on my left hand gave me a sense of security and hope, but the year ahead seemed interminable. Letters flew back and forth on a daily basis. Occasionally a package replaced a letter.

Valentine's Day 1953 — a difficult day to be without a loved one under any circumstances. But when I arrived home from class that afternoon, there in the foyer, amidst the usual inviting array of mail, lay a well-traveled package tied with brown string. It was addressed to me, with that familiar name in the upper left-hand corner. He remembered! As the outer layers gave way, the enclosed box appeared, carefully gift-wrapped in silver and gold flecked white paper and tied with wide gold ribbon. U of I colors! Inside I found a complete place-setting of the sterling pattern we had selected together, with these words carefully tucked in-between the layers of tissue paper:

Dear Pat,

I looked over a lot of cards designed for the occasion, but they just didn't have "it." Even tried the old last resort, moldy poetry, but didn't have the heart to submit the results.

It's not easy to try to transmit the love I have for you by mail — yet I like to try to let you know how I feel. Right now the most noticeable effect is the loneliness that comes from knowing that the real main spring in my life is so far away. Beneath that, there's great pride in knowing that you love me, and boundless faith in you and your abilities. Sometimes I wonder how I could be so fortunate to find and win so wonderful a girl as you.

But for now, all this must go through the mail. I can't help but feel that it loses a little in the process, so I wanted to take advantage of this occasion to say how very much I love you in a slightly special way.

I kinda like to think that this silver is a bit symbolic of the bond we have between us, Pat. It's bright. It's new. It's beautiful, and it's something that will last a lifetime and gain in meaning and value all the way.

Here's to you, Pat, with all the love in my heart.

Don

What an awesome gift. What a heartwarming note. He loved me. I loved him. Suddenly Valentine's Day didn't seem so lonely, and the miles between us didn't matter.

Chapter Three

In order to complete my last year of college by May —
when I knew Don would finish his current assignment with the
Air Force — I took accelerated classes and correspondence
courses, and buried myself in books that spring. It was worth
the effort, because, in late May of 1953, we had a simple
wedding ceremony at my parents' home in California.

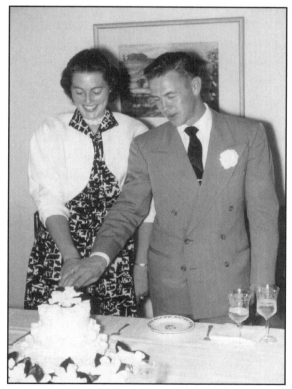

May 21, 1953
San Carlos,
California

We spent a glorious two-week honeymoon roaming the coastal roads between San Francisco and Los Angeles; then in early June Don received his new orders. He was assigned to the Far East, with no final destination designated.

So we parted once again. I had no choice but to live with my parents, work in the city, and wait to hear where Don would be stationed. I began the familiar routine of checking for mail each evening. Days went by, and after what seemed an eternity, finally two letters arrived! Being the "good" daughter, I dutifully ate dinner and visited with my parents before making time to be alone that night. Then I retired to my room, carefully shut the bedroom door, and was soon grinning at, and warmed by, Don's closing words in the first envelope that I opened.

"You can't imagine how proudly I wear this gold ring," he wrote. "It looks nice, fits, and more important, it's there to stay! I miss you more than ever, and love you with all my heart."

That gold ring hadn't always been there to stay. On our honeymoon, we camped out one evening under the majestic redwoods at Big Basin. Don's new wedding ring was a bit too large for his finger, and as we crawled into our double sleeping bag that night, it slipped off! We were not very well equipped for camping — we didn't even have a flashlight — and had anyone been observing, we would have made a comical sight as we groped around in the dark on our hands and knees trying to find the elusive ring. We finally found that precious circle of gold, and at the first jewelers we could find, we had it sized to fit properly!

Don's second letter shared the news that he had been assigned to an Air Force base near Tokyo, and that he would be in Japan until August 1954.

August of 1954! Separated for another year?

No.

If Don was going to be in Japan, I was going to be in Japan!

I began searching for information. How does one go about getting from San Francisco to Tokyo? Not an easy task, I discovered. My parents were supportive, but for many in 1953, the idea of a 21-year-old female boarding a ship and heading for Japan to meet a young Air Force Lieutenant was not viewed as a wise thing to do — married or not married. The Korean War was winding down, and an armistice was signed in late July — but due to the unrest in that part of the world, Japan was not considered a safe place for a young American female.

Following Don to Japan was not only unwise, said some people, but also probably an unobtainable goal. Travel from the U.S. to Japan was expensive. I needed to take not only my personal belongings, but also any household goods we would need for the entire year, was the overwhelming message. Going by freighter seemed to be the only option. Obtaining space on a freighter was not easy to do. Obtaining the proper visa was challenging. If I went over on my own, the Air Force might not pay for my passage back to the States. Decent and affordable off-base housing was almost unheard of. Living expenses in the Tokyo area were considered prohibitive. "Wives don't like it here," Don was told.

On and on went the reasons for not going. Nevertheless, Don diligently saved his paycheck and searched for potential housing in Japan, while I set aside each penny I earned to pay for transportation, and used every ounce of ingenuity and determination I possessed to get there.

After working my way through the seemingly endless amounts of paperwork, frustrating delays, and innumerable road blocks, I sent Don a telegram.

"I can leave on a freighter on September 26. Please advise."

His response came back quickly: "Pack your best sense of humor and come on over."

"I will find a place for us to live," he vowed in the letter that arrived a week and a half later.

And on the twenty-sixth day of September, I was on my way! With a steamer trunk full of clothes, several packing cases filled with household goods, a passport, a visa, a sense of accomplishment, and high hopes, I boarded a small freighter headed north for a brief stop at Campbell River, British Columbia, and then on to Yokohama, Japan.

The next 19 days were quite an education for a young woman just out of college in 1953. There were five other wives aboard the ship, all en route to meet their men. My roommate, Julie, and I were the youngest, and the least experienced in many ways, we were soon to discover.

As we crossed over numerous time zones, my own sense of time soon became warped. There were times when I would be prowling the ship at strange hours. On cloudless nights, unbelievable numbers of stars decorated the broad, dark sky. They were brilliant and clear, as they sparkled over the vast expanse of ocean upon which we seemed to move ever so slowly. I was filled with awe. It was amazing to me that it was possible to find one's way across that immense body of water, with only twinkling stars as guides.

The small crew of seamen was very friendly, and quite accommodating! Johnny, the fellow who befriended me, shared his expertise about navigating the high seas, using maps, charts, and a gyroscope. Eventually it became quite clear, even to my inexperienced head, that he would be happy to share other kinds of expertise as well. On one occasion, the rather openended comment was made that if I were not married, he would be, ah, very interested . . .

I had been observing that several friendships seemed to be developing aboard the ship . . .

One rough and stormy night, a time when experienced travelers would have known to stay in their cabins, Julie and I went exploring. As the ship heaved and rolled and rain splattered all around us, we laughingly inched our way around the deck, hanging on to the attached railings by the cabins for dear life. Together, we cautiously peered through a small porthole on the opposite side of the ship. As we stared in fascination, we quickly confirmed our suspicions. "Friendships" were indeed being cultivated in some of the staterooms!

Amazingly, we arrived back in our small room intact. How easily the two of us could have been swept right off that narrow deck by the driving wind and rain. In our naivete, we had not even given the imminent danger a thought.

We found our stateroom in chaos — several suitcases and a metal wastebasket crashed back and forth from one side of the small room to the other. When I released my grip on the door handle, I suddenly found myself on the seat of my pants sliding across the floor along with the other objects. After the initial surprise, I soon began roaring with laughter — a great opportunity to release the tension from our on-deck escapade! Julie, at first a bit hesitant, soon joined in.

Ah, yes. An educational experience, that sea voyage. And how young we were . . .

After bouncing around on those rough fall seas for 19 days, our little ship finally arrived in the calm waters of Tokyo Bay. As we moved slowly toward the loading dock in Yokohama, my eyes eagerly scanned the waiting forms in the distance. He was almost hidden behind the wooden pilings, but I finally spotted the one I had crossed the ocean to be with. It seemed to take forever for the ship to slowly jockey into position and dock, for the gangplank to be set in place, for the line of waiting people there on the dock to arrive on deck. Then suddenly, in an unbelievably magical moment, we were in each other's arms. What joy! What ecstasy!

And what excitement, to walk hand in hand across that pier in Yokohama, Japan, toward the waiting Air Force truck and our new life together. The exhilaration was overwhelming. It wasn't until we finally curled up together that first night that the pent-up emotion of the last months, and the unequaled elation of actually being there with Don in that far-away country truly caught up with me. I quietly dissolved into tears of joy.

Our first year of marriage was an enchanting one. We lived off-base in a little house in a small complex where several American families were living. We eventually obtained some pieces of western furniture from the base, but our first nights were spent on the bedroom's rice mat floor, with the typical futons spread out for our bed. The low doorways quickly helped us learn to duck each time we went from room to room. There was no central heating, and we learned to survive with one small oil space heater.

I soon found a secretarial job on the base. During the weekends, we went exploring. Don always had his camera in his hand or slung over his shoulder, and he became extremely skilled at capturing, on film, glimpses of what we saw with our eyes. We walked and walked. We rode the buses, the trains, and then bicycles, which we purchased for added mobility. There were so many things to see, hear, smell, taste, and experience!

The trains were modern, immaculate, often extremely crowded — and very punctual. When we wanted to sightsee in Tokyo, we took one train from the little village near Don's base, and changed to a different line at Shinjuku Station. One Saturday morning, we hurried from one part of the station to another to catch the connecting train. We stood on the platform with the other waiting passengers. The train pulled up, opened its doors, and people streamed in. Don preceded me. I stepped back briefly to let an elderly Japanese woman move onto the waiting train, and all of a sudden the doors slammed shut! There I stood on the platform, with Don wedged in with the others on the train as it rapidly pulled away! We shared a brief look of shock, and he was gone. Don told me later that the people jammed together in the packed car watched the whole scenario, and erupted with understanding laughter and recognition as they observed our plight.

In the meantime, I stood wondering just what I should do! Our knowledge of the Japanese language was limited. We had formulated no plans for any separation. Would Don get off at the next station? Would he go on to the main train station in downtown Tokyo where we were originally headed? Another train pulled up. I got on, eyed each stop, did not see Don, stayed put, and was greatly relieved to see Don and his familiar grin there to greet me when I stepped off the train and onto the platform in Tokyo's busy downtown terminal!

Some weekends we rode the trains to other cities such as Kamakura and Kyoto. We marveled at the Great Buddha, the huge torii (arches erected on the approach to every Shinto shrine), the shrines themselves, the beautiful Japanese gardens. We traveled to remote villages on skiing and hiking trips, sipped Ocha at local tea houses, and sampled dishes of all kinds. Tempura and sukiyaki rapidly became our favorites, although mastering the art of always eating those tasty meals with chopsticks provided a bit of a challenge!

Few Japanese homes had tubs and showers as we know them. Large community baths and smaller "intimate" baths for couples could be found in the cities, in tiny villages, and in many hotels. Everyone would wash on the adjoining deck, then soak together in the steaming bath. We weren't quite ready to participate in the community bath, but thoroughly enjoyed lounging in the piping hot water of the smaller, private ones!

Our train trip to Kyoto provided some very special memories from that year in Japan.

Early one Saturday morning, our train moved quickly out of Tokyo's main station and the downtown area. The clean and shining rail car wound its way through the low buildings on the outskirts of the city, and we watched with fascination as the panorama of the nearby countryside began to stretch before our eyes.

We passed miles and miles of rice fields, some on flat land, some built like steps up the steep hillsides. Men and women worked those fields — many wearing wide-brimmed rice-straw hats for protection from the sun. Weathered wooden houses, with their typical wide and open front decks were perched on the edge of that land. In front of the houses, we saw women washing clothes in large wooden containers. They had garments strung out on long bamboo poles to dry, with poles going through the sleeves of a shirt, or through the legs of pants. We saw men and women of all ages carrying heavy loads evenly balanced on either end of bamboo poles, or carefully balanced on their backs. Some were walking, some were on bicycles. We saw children playing near the houses or walking along the road, some carrying smaller ones on their backs. We waved, and with huge grins, those young people eagerly waved back.

We opened up paper lunch bags that held our tuna fish sandwiches, carrots, apples, and cookies. Our fellow travelers opened up their meals — perhaps consisting of rice, vegetables, fish, and rice cakes — that had been neatly wrapped in squares of colorful cloth.

While we were eating, the train stopped at a busy little station. We joined the many passengers who raised the car's windows to make purchases from the vendors who moved up and down the wooden platform, calling out their wares. We were well aware that one should not drink unboiled water, but knew the bottled drinks were considered safe. We laughed with those vendors as we struggled to understand one another, and as Don and I scrambled to produce the proper currency. Just as the train moved slowly away from the station, we succeeded in purchasing two carbonated orange drinks to go with our sandwiches!

Eventually we arrived in Kyoto, also called Heian-kyo (the city of peace), and noted as the "Spiritual home of all Japanese people" in one of our brochures. We found a small hotel near the train station, then set out to explore that enchanting city. We took a bus tour, then walked and walked.

Kyoto was known for its magnificent shrines, temples and torii, lovely gardens, tea houses, tea ceremonies, and colorful festivals. Many of the shrines and temples were immense, with ornate carving and stunning architecture. The exquisite gardens, with their winding walkways laid with small white stones, intricately-trimmed pine trees, and ponds with small arched bridges that led from one little island to another, were all something to behold. The age and beauty, the stillness of those shrines, temples, and gardens, filled us with a sense of awe and wonder, a sense of peace.

That evening, after a marvelous tempura dinner in a small restaurant near the hotel, we set out walking once again. Kyoto was so much like any city in the U.S. on a Saturday night, yet so very different. The main thoroughfare was filled with walkers, cyclers with their clanging bells, a few cars, music, and bright lights. Fascinating sights, sounds, and aromas surrounded us.

With the security of Don's hand in mine, I felt no fear in those cities in 1953. We found the concerns of those in the States who had qualms about an American's safety in Japan to be unfounded. We were always greeted by warm, friendly, and helpful people.

We came to a small alleyway that led off to the right, then curved around to the left. It seemed quieter, intriguing, and inviting.

Down the narrow walkway we strolled on that pleasant spring evening. As the path became narrower, the shops became smaller, the lights dimmer, and the sounds even quieter. We passed tiny tea shops, small restaurants, several little specialty shops. We moved past a young Japanese couple, also hand in hand, and exchanged understanding smiles.

On and on we went. The walkway seemed to become more and more narrow. Then suddenly it ended. A tiny, dimly-lit tea shop was on our left. Oriental music drifted from an alluring bath house on the right. How could we resist?

With gestures, our limited Japanese, and the help of pictures in the brochures on the small desk, we soon found ourselves settled in an "intimate bath for partners." We carefully washed, rinsed with the small wooden buckets that sat on the wooden deck beside the tub, then slowly, and very cautiously, slipped into the steaming water. As Westerners, we weren't quite addicted to the same high temperatures that the Japanese so loved. But what a delightful, relaxing experience the hot baths always were.

That night we lounged in the tub until we found ourselves falling asleep . . . then reluctantly climbed out and struggled to pull our clothes onto our warm bodies. We moved across the narrow walkway to the little teahouse, savored a cup of green tea and several tasty rice cakes, then slowly wound our way back to the main street.

When we finally found ourselves on the busy avenue once again, and on our way back to our hotel, we grinned at one another. We could have stayed on the bustling sidewalk, not taken that "walkway less traveled," and never known what lay beyond. Something caught our eye, captured our imagination — and how glad we were that we took a step here, a turn there, away from the path we had been walking. We discovered and experienced things we could never have imagined, things that could not be seen from where we were, had we not dared to step off into the unknown.

I have thought about that experience many times over the years, when fear of the unknown has threatened to keep me from moving out to explore new horizons. It serves as a reminder to always evaluate fears, to seek to be open to new directions, new experiences, new ideas — a reminder that pleasure, beauty, joy, a sense of peace or fulfillment can be found in what may be considered unexpected places.

With mixed emotions of regret at leaving Japan, and eagerness to return to the U.S., we pulled out of Japanese waters

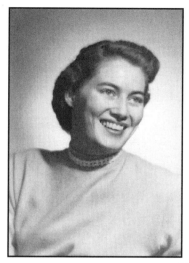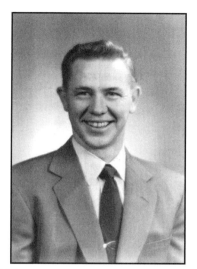

1954

in August of 1954, sailed across the Pacific, under the Golden Gate, and into San Francisco Bay together. Don had completed his tour of duty with the Air Force. He was scheduled to return to the corporation's training program, which allowed a young engineer to spend several months at a number of different plants in order to gain diverse exposure within the organization. His first three-month assignment was in western New York. We bought a nifty little white 1950 Chevrolet in the Bay Area, and headed East. The assignments that followed took us to Kentucky, Massachusetts and Pennsylvania.

What a unique opportunity those short assignments provided. Not only were they great opportunities for Don to work in a variety of departments within the company, but also they allowed us to explore new cities, see new and different parts of our vast country. In each location I looked for, and always found, a secretarial or office job of some kind.

Again, we found many ways to enjoy weekends, and took full advantage of our free time! We found lakes, streams, and ocean beaches for swimming. We went hiking, camping, and skiing in the mountains of New England and Pennsylvania. We roamed through museums and parks in Boston, New York City, and Philadelphia. We dined in exotic restaurants, "Hole-in-the-wall" restaurants — and carried our bag lunches. We went to Boston Pops concerts. On various weekend trips into New York City we saw *My Fair Lady*, *Can-Can*, *The Most Happy Fella*, and *Damn Yankees*. We took the Circle Line Tour around Manhattan. We visited college friends who had settled in the East, and on longer vacations drove up and down the coast between Canada and Florida, stopping in many places that had once been only names for us.

Those were very special years we enjoyed as two during the early part of our marriage.

But there did come a time when we hoped for a family. It was in Philadelphia that we became the proud parents of our first child, a daughter, Sandra Kaye, who was born in January 1959.

That fall we moved back to the state of New York, where Don accepted a permanent position with the company. He joined an elite group of top-notch engineers dealing with analyses and equipment applications in electrical systems. This group was highly respected within the company, and by

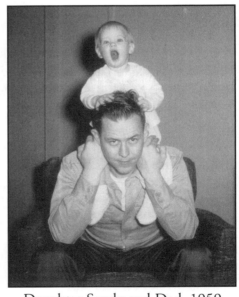

Daughter Sandy and Dad, 1959

clients with whom they worked outside the organization. It was a unit made up of 18 to 20 individuals — a close-knit, knowledgeable group, working together and sharing expertise. The overall atmosphere was one of cooperation and camaraderie, and Don was excited and enthusiastic about being part of that outstanding operation.

For a few years his job was rewarding and satisfying, but things began to change drastically for him in early 1962. Don started reporting to a man who was very different from his previous manager. This individual could be very brusque, controlling, opinionated, and vindictive. Often his pattern was to "put down" anyone working under him. There were others in the unit who worked hard at steering clear of this man, but Don's position and job requirements did not allow him that option. We spent long hours talking, as Don vented his anger and frustration. We were both aware that not much could be done to change the situation, but we had learned that feeling free to share our feelings and talk out loud about something that bothered us, led to our ability to see a problem more clearly, and often to thoughts and ideas that we could not have come to alone.

In spite of the fact that these years were a difficult and stressful period in Don's career, we were able to maintain happy and fun times in our home and personal lives. In 1963, our second daughter, Lisa Suzanne, joined our small family. We

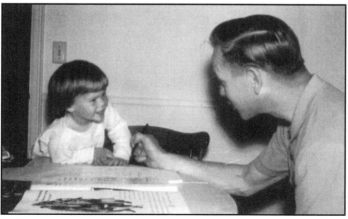

Daughter Lisa and Dad, 1964

enjoyed being parents, and were delighted to have another daughter.

Don was a wonderful dad. And how proud he was of his daughters. He helped take care of them when they were babies, played with them as they grew, fixed their broken toys, read them stories, helped them with their homework, taught them his love of running by running with them, and always had a ready listening ear, and caring heart.

I, too, appreciated Don's listening ear and caring heart. When we shared our thoughts, feelings, hopes, and dreams — whether we talked as we cleaned up after dinner or spent an evening in front of the fire — I always knew that he was listening with his heart, with his whole being.

One evening, with a straight face and familiar twinkle in his eye, he quietly slipped an 8½ x 11 piece of paper across the dinner table. A large picture took up the entire sheet. It was a carefully drawn depiction of an elephant! Its trunk was lowered, then curled up at the end, and clutched a small sign that read, "Please Don't Eat The Elephants."

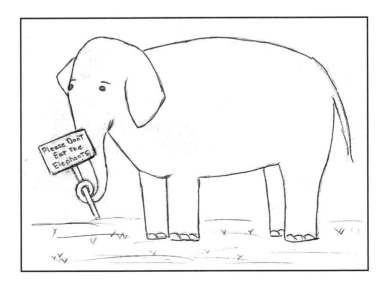

I scanned the picture, and sheepishly grinned with recognition. I knew exactly what his simple sketch meant, exactly what he was trying to help me remember.

The night before I had been "bending" his ear, struggling with some problem that seemed monumental at the time. I was attempting to deal with whatever the challenge was by looking at the whole scenario . . . eating the whole "elephant" . . . and it was overwhelming me. I was well-practiced and quite skilled at this endeavor.

Don was well-practiced and extremely skilled at listening and trying to help me keep my perspective. We both chuckled over his simple sketch, and over the years it served as a reminder to try to take any challenge we were concerned about one "bite," one step, at a time. Sometimes we remembered, but more often than not, I was the one who forgot!

Don was not afraid to express his emotions with hugs, with spoken words, with words on paper. He was not afraid to tell us he loved us, and with great regularity and deep feeling he did so. There was a hug and kiss for everyone when he arrived home from work. There were carefully chosen cards for every occasion, loving and humorous notes tacked up on the refrigerator when he left for work in the morning, and special notes and cards that arrived in the mail when he was out of town. Before he left for work each morning, he would retrieve the newspaper from the front porch and leave it on the kitchen counter. Often I would find "Don loves Pat!" carefully printed in large letters right above the daily headlines.

He was very "at home" in the kitchen — often helping fix dinner, and always helping with the cleanup. He enjoyed baking scrumptious homemade bread and delicious pies of all kinds, which all four of us eagerly devoured. Don and I would clean and de-vein mounds of raw shrimp and cut up all kinds of fresh vegetables for tempura — then it was Don who prepared a delectable batter and fried the tasty morsels one by one in our electric skillet. Whether it was just the four of us around our table or a dinner shared with friends, that delicious meal was always a marvelous treat — a meal we had loved in Japan, and one our daughters learned to enjoy as much as we did.

And he was always there to do things as a family. Sometimes we took the girls on "mystery car trips" — not telling them where we were going. They were always excited, and still remember those excursions with pleasure. On other weekends and vacations the four of us went swimming, picnicking, canoeing, and camping at some of the beautiful cool, clear lakes that can be found in the state of New York. We went sledding and skiing. We drove to Maine to spend summer vacations in Ogunquit, to Pennsylvania to spend weekends in the center of Philadelphia, flew West to see our families.

These years were filled with love and memorable times, in spite of the challenges Don faced at work.

Then during the mid-sixties, there were changes in his department that held new hope. Another shuffle in management took place that resulted in an entirely different atmosphere for everyone, especially for Don. I remember so well the sighs of relief we shared, and the glint of excitement in his eyes, when he was finally out from under the previous manager and once again working in a comfortable, satisfying, stimulating environment.

For the next fifteen years, Don's career was rewarding and productive. He authored technical papers, presented them at conferences, gave seminars, taught classes, mentored young engineers in his unit, and had many opportunities to grow and develop technically, professionally, and personally. He enjoyed his work, he enjoyed the people with whom he worked, within and outside the company, and he was held in high regard by his colleagues. However, because of Don's sensitive nature, the stress of the assignment in the early sixties continued to rear its ugly head. The fear of being judged inadequate again remained an underlying concern that he could not dislodge.

Chapter Four

When was it that I first noticed changes in Don? What were the warnings that began to register in my mind? I think there were little things that began to puzzle, and sometimes irritate me, but they are as difficult to pinpoint now as they were then. I do remember that there came a time when I realized he seemed very different from the handsome young college student, and later the dashing Air Force officer, who wrote me the cherished poems and letters of the early 1950s. I knew that everyone and everything changes . . . I was definitely no longer the same romantic young woman who fell in love, married Don Miller, and followed him to Japan and beyond. But the changes I noticed in Don didn't seem like "normal" changes.

In trying to recall what things I noticed and when I noticed them, our twenty-fifth year begins to stand out as a difficult one. As we approached that silver anniversary in 1978, I remember wondering if I really wanted to continue in the marriage — an idea I never would have believed I would consider. Slowly some of the reasons for such a thought have filtered into my consciousness.

The changes in Don had definitely been gradual and subtle. His eagerness to try new things, his enthusiasm for life, and his hope for the future seemed to have completely disappeared. Even his delightful sense of humor didn't surface very often. He had just turned fifty that year, but dealing with everyday affairs, and keeping up with the challenges at work, appeared to take all of his mental energy.

I found myself feeling more and more frustrated with Don, with our relationship, and with his moving through life almost by rote. And he seemed frustrated with himself! I remember him saying that he was the world's first "mechanical man" and talking about his sense of plodding, of living in a deep blue funk.

The loss of a precious stone, and a letter from Don, contributed to the turning point in my thinking during that challenging year.

We came out of a movie theater one evening, and with panic, I suddenly realized that the center diamond was missing from my engagement ring. Don and I hurried back into the theater, told the manager our story, and soon two young ushers joined us as we crawled around and under the seats we had used. But there was no trace of that little stone.

That evening, I set my ring with its gaping hole on the dark brown place mat in the center of the kitchen table. Perhaps Don would see it and replace the diamond.

Weeks passed, and the ring remained on our table.

It may have been motionless — my thoughts were not.

I had lost my diamond, and we seemed to have lost some of the magic and promise that gem symbolized. It occurred to me that I had four options. I could continue to dwell on all of the things in our marriage that frustrated me . . . and continue to make comments to Don about that frustration. I could set aside the desires, hopes, and dreams I held for the two of us, and be content with the rather humdrum existence that recently had seemed to satisfy Don. I could leave. Or . . . I could change my attitude, and work harder at finding ways to bring more good things into our lives.

A letter from Don on the day of our anniversary that year recaptured my heart, resealed our love — and our marriage.

Dear Pat,

Cards are hard to find — we have said that more times than we can remember. And what card can say what is really inside? For me, the message inside seems so hard to express. So — I retreat to ready-made messages, which at best only point in the direction I might go. And always, they stop short of saying what I would like to say.

I love you so much. I write the words on cards and notes and say them to you, but I want you to know that it is deep and real. I respect you and the honesty in relationships you have, and your ability to say what needs to be said. I have confidence that these qualities and others are the basis for progress to something new in our relationship. I do not want to cut and sever what can be untangled, strengthened and made better, and hope for a stronger and closer relationship between us in the future.

I love you very much.

Don

I took my engagement ring to the jewelers myself, priced diamonds, and decided their cost was an extravagance. A display of birth stones provided inspiration. I would replace the diamond with my August birth stone. I would put something of myself into the ring, and more of myself into our marriage to make it work.

Looking back, I am overwhelmed with gratitude that I did not choose the option to leave. In spite of my frustrations, I was not ready to walk away from the loyal and loving man who had loved me so long and so well, who loved me still, and whom I really knew I loved deeply.

I was the one who made changes — mostly in my attitude and expectations. The things about Don that frustrated me did not change . . . and now I understand why they did not. But he steadfastly remained the same high-class individual, continued to love me, be loyal to me, and reflect his great respect for me, in spite of the disease that may well have been silently creeping up on him as early as 1978.

A few years later, changes at work added to the stress Don seemed to be experiencing. He had always found great satisfaction in the consulting and technical application work he did, thoroughly enjoyed his involvement with people within and outside the company, and was very grateful to be working once again in a comfortable environment. But in 1979 and 1980, Don and others in his unit found that the load they each carried began to slowly increase, and the pace of the entire operation seemed to become more rapid.

Then in 1981, the group's commercial/pricing person unexpectedly left the company, and Don was asked to pick up the slack in that area. His manager thought the additional responsibilities would not be too heavy, and that they would not interfere too much with Don's normal workload. Don wasn't so sure, but decided he should not turn the request down.

Unfortunately, shortly after the decision was made, circumstances within the unit changed again. The requirements of the job became 100 percent commercial, and Don was soon buried in charts and numbers connected with pricing. There was no time for the consulting and project work he enjoyed so much.

After struggling for a while, Don formally requested that he be relieved of the pricing work as soon as possible. But it took over two years to find a suitable replacement for the commercial position — and those years were difficult ones.

Don was finally able to hand the pricing responsibilities over to someone else. But his frustrations increased when he found it difficult to help customers with their problems, when the ability to meet the requirements of some of the projects he was assigned eluded him, or when it took more time than he felt it should to finish a job. And he found himself completely mystified by the new personal computers his fellow engineers were finding so helpful in their technical work. In an effort to keep up, he spent many evenings working at home. Moving back to his original position also meant working under a different manager. This man was a fine engineer and long-time friend, but he was far more skilled as an engineer than he was as a manager. We learned later that during the next few years inputs from various sources began to hint that the quality of Don's project work was slipping. However friendship, and the hesitancy to deal with an awkward situation, seemed to have kept this good friend-turned-manager from talking with Don about it.

Qualified system application engineers became more difficult to locate. The unit grew smaller and smaller, as colleagues began to retire and were not replaced. The workload each person carried continued to be a heavy one, and in their attempts to keep up, everyone began to work alone more often. The previously close-knit group had enjoyed sharing and discussing ideas — both personal and job related — and that sense of camaraderie seemed to slowly slip away. Don began to feel isolated — which added to his feelings of inadequacy.

All of his life he had been an extremely conscientious person. The fact that the computers seemed to almost frighten him, and that he made no attempt to take classes or find some way to learn more about them or catch up technically, puzzled others in his unit. Looking back, it is easier to understand that the lack of action on Don's part was another indication of the unseen forces that were pulling him downhill.

As I thought about these events, I began to remember other things that I had noticed that seemed out-of-character for this sharp and intelligent man.

Gradually Don began to rely on me increasingly for map reading and navigating on strange roads, and later, on familiar roads. His driving became more and more "sloppy."

I began to notice his growing inability to remember where we were in familiar malls, where we had come in, how to get back out the same entrance, and how to find the car. But aren't there occasions when many of us struggle with these problems? I didn't make much of the observations at the time.

He had trouble balancing the checkbook at home, and checks were returned unsigned. The clock radio "didn't work." My favorite "fix-it" man around the house found it more and more difficult to remedy the problems that arise in the lives of homeowners. Equipment he was to take on trips for projects at work "wouldn't function properly," and each one he received as a replacement seemed to have problems as well . . . His concern about spending so many hours on each job he was assigned deepened, and the amount of work he brought home increased. He was unbelievably frustrated, and so was I. Neither of us understood these changes, and I didn't know what to do nor how to help.

I remember when he was on a business trip to California in the mid-eighties, and planned to fly to Idaho to visit his family before coming home. When he was at the San Francisco airport, he called, sounding confused, frustrated, and tired. He had been unable to locate the right gate. He had missed his plane, and was trying to work out new arrangements.

His brother-in-law met him at the Boise airport, and told me later that Don was visibly shaken and upset when he got off the plane. He suggested that Don join him in a small coffee shop there in the airport so that they could have a bite to eat, hoping that the opportunity to talk and relax together might help. It did. But after that visit, his sister and her family shared later that they, too, had noticed subtle changes. He seemed like a much older man than they remembered — not quite like the fun-loving, light-hearted, enthusiastic individual the family had known for so long.

In January 1988, Don's troubles became unavoidably conspicuous. He began a study for one of his regular clients in an area of expertise in which he had always been highly skilled. I could tell that he was having trouble completing the study and meeting the deadline for its presentation, which was scheduled to take place at a good-sized conference in another state.

When Don stood to address the group, his concern about the quality of his material, his confusion and growing panic about the whole situation, were painfully obvious. The entire scene involved with the presentation was a disaster, with no one able to understand why this experienced, highly-respected engineer was struggling so to deal with the technical aspects of the study, its presentation, and even with finding his way to the proper meeting room on several occasions.

I went on that particular trip with Don. In the airport on the way home, I was filled with a deep sense of foreboding. I knew that something was very wrong.

We returned home, and the next months became increasingly difficult for Don. He continued to have a great deal of trouble handling jobs that never would have been a problem for him in the past. Yet with a herculean effort, he continued to struggle along that spring and summer of 1988.

One afternoon in August, his manager asked him to come into his office for a meeting. When he walked in, he was suddenly confronted by not one person, but two people. There sat his manager and long-time friend, and beside him at a large table sat the young man to whom they both reported. The two men just sat . . . waiting.

Both of these men were well aware that Don's skills and overall performance at work were slipping drastically. Although I learned later the two of them had often discussed that reality for at least a year and a half, they had never approached Don about it. To their credit, when Don went for his yearly company physical that spring, they covertly asked the doctor to see if he could find anything that might account for the difficulties Don was having. The physician reported that he saw nothing amiss.

It must have been challenging for them to know what to do about the whole situation, but it is not easy for me to comprehend their choice of action. They had decided to simply confront him, on that August afternoon of 1988.

Don was very aware that he continued to have problems with jobs he was assigned. But he had no idea how significantly the quality of his work was deteriorating. Suddenly, now came not only extensive, but also extremely critical and chastising remarks about the study he had done in January, and profuse accusations of inadequate and improper work on many other projects over the last 17 months.

The abrupt two-on-one session was followed by a long letter which appeared on Don's desk early the next morning:

Mr. D. F. Miller:

Confirming the discussion we had today, we are concerned that your performance has deteriorated substantially over the last several years, and most noticeably over the last six or eight months. We are concerned about this because as business managers in this organization we cannot tolerate substandard performance; it is incumbent on us to take corrective action as appropriate to the circumstances. We want you to know, however, that we are also greatly concerned on the personal level because of our long association, friendship, and respect. This is why we have encouraged you to carefully review your situation and seek help to identify and resolve the problem.

There have been a number of specific customer instances which illustrate the extent of the problem. In each case, an isolated view would suggest that you might have been the "fall guy" in a bad situation usually resulting from the actions of others. However, in total, the trend suggests a deterioration of your abilities in the technical, administrative, and customer relations aspects of your job.

More fundamentally, we have sensed a growing discomfort with technology and a tendency toward disorientation and forgetfulness. Given your continued dedication to both the company and your job, we are concerned that your performance problem may reflect an underlying personal problem. For this reason we suggest that you seek help through the company's employee assistance program.

Don, in pointing out this problem to you, we are doing a necessary, but unpleasant part of our jobs.

The next step is up to you.

The next two pages carefully detailed the problems they perceived, situation by situation, job by job.

They didn't know what was wrong . . .

None of us did.

They didn't know how to handle the situation. I know they regretted their actions later.

Most of us make errors in judgment over the years — it seems almost impossible not to . . .

But I can't even imagine how Don truly felt as he sat across from those two men that afternoon, or how he felt as he read those words in their letter the next morning.

Ever since we'd returned from Japan in 1954, he had given his all to a company that had his complete loyalty, to a career that was much of his life and the basis of his identity. The unexpected derogatory remarks, the inordinate number of claims of poor performance, the chastisement, must have been an unbelievable blow, must have hurt him deeply.

When Don came home the evening after the meeting, he seemed to be almost in shock. His eyes were glazed, and as he struggled to share what had happened, it was obvious that this kind, gentle, and dedicated man was completely devastated.

We wrote a letter in his defense, and asked that it accompany their letter in his personnel file. Over the next months we did seek help from the company's employee assistance program, and consulted with a variety of doctors within our local medical community.

Our search led us to a man who specialized in neurology. He requested that we have a broad range of tests taken — including an Electroencephalogram (EEG), Magnetic Resonance Imagery (MRI), blood work, and psychological tests. One afternoon in October, we went to his office to get the test results. That was when we received the doctor's blunt, cruel assessment.

Perhaps I was in denial, as the neurologist had declared. But considering all I knew about Don Miller, about all that had been part of his job situation over recent years, it seemed plausible that severe depression, or something like post-traumatic syndrome or pseudo-dementia, could be causing the problems he was experiencing. How could he possibly have Alzheimer's disease? In my mind, that illness had always been connected with afflictions later in life, problems that as a young woman I remembered being labeled "senile dementia." Don was only 59! And just "yesterday" we were 22 and 24, newly married, and spending our first year together in Japan. I became determined to prove that doctor wrong.

In January 1989, I called to make an appointment for a complete evaluation for Don at a well-known hospital and diagnostic clinic. I had made many inquiries about where there were clinics that investigated medical problems, and chose this one because of its fine reputation. And there was another plus. Our younger daughter, Lisa, had become a Registered Occupational Therapist (O.T.R.), and was currently working at a psychiatric hospital in the same city. The availability of her support, and the inputs and suggestions from a highly-respected doctor friend of hers, made it seem not only an excellent, but a logical choice.

After extensive testing, that outstanding group of medical people felt that 75 percent of the problem could be due to stress, and that 25 percent was something for which they could not account. They were extremely knowledgeable, helpful, and supportive people, and Don and I came home feeling both relief and hope. They made a few suggestions that they felt might alleviate some of the pressure at work, suggested that Don work on plans for his retirement years, and that we find a good psychiatrist in our area to work with him.

But the local psychiatrist with whom we consulted looked at the records we had accumulated, spent a few sessions with Don, and decided that he agreed with the original Alzheimer's diagnosis. He met with me alone, told me he did not feel that either therapy or antidepressants would help, and with great empathy warned me that there was a long road ahead. Then he quietly suggested that I might want to consider a divorce, on paper only, to protect myself financially.

"No," I thought on the way home. "I don't want to consider even a 'paper' divorce." No matter what lay ahead, for me that idea was not an acceptable one. The idea of separating had crossed my mind in 1978, and been rejected. Now divorce was something I didn't even want to consider — in any form.

And in spite of hearing an Alzheimer's diagnosis once again, I was simply not willing to accept the idea.

I researched, read, asked questions, and was beginning to understand a little about the illness. At that point in time, it was not something that could be accurately determined while the patient was living. Alzheimer's disease could only be confirmed by an autopsy. Medical people came to a diagnosis of "Possible" or "Probable" Alzheimer's disease through the process of elimination. And, there was a form of the illness that was called "early onset" Alzheimer's.

Although the group at the clinic had ruled out many things, they had not been ready to "label" Don's problems. I was not ready to label them either.

Over the next months, we talked with other medical people in our area. It seemed to me there was a tendency to take a quick look at the records that we had accumulated and just say, "Yes, your husband has Alzheimer's disease." I desperately wanted to find someone who would take a careful and open-minded look to see if there was any possibility that the stress and hurts Don had experienced at work during the last few years could be connected with his problems. It seemed to me that it would be worth at least trying an antidepressant.

I sought information about several less conventional approaches, and soon discovered that there are people in many unusual areas of expertise who feel they can do great and wonderful things for someone who may have Alzheimer's disease. We tried a few of those unconventional approaches, and walked away from one that definitely had an air of quackery about it.

I began to realize that we desperately needed a break, that we needed to do something just for fun. One of the suggestions from the doctors at the clinic had been for Don to request that he work under a different manager. That was accomplished, but because of his shrinking abilities, the job situation continued to be a challenging one.

The stress was getting to both of us. Even though I had traveled with Don on business trips in the last year or two, and we had taken several trips to see our daughters in the South, now it seemed important to take a real vacation for just the two of us.

With Don's confusion worsening, I felt a familiar spot not too far from home would be the best choice. In the fall of 1989, we headed for our favorite lake in upstate New York, one where we had spent many wonderful times camping, swimming, and canoeing.

On this occasion, we spent five extra-special days in an attractive and well-furnished log cabin beside the lake. It was nestled among the pine trees, yet had a spectacular view of both the water and the mountains. The early autumn weather was perfect — warm and sunny, with clear blue skies. How we enjoyed the clean fresh air and the smell of the pines, as we roamed the many hiking trails. We sat on a huge rock near our cabin, and listened to the sound of water lapping onto the shore. We watched the sun set behind the backdrop of the mountains across the often still waters of early evening. Later, as we sat beside a cozy fire in the rustic fireplace, I read aloud from our books of short stories by Mark Twain and O. Henry.

In spite of the fact that there were moments when Don was confused or struggling with anger and frustration about his situation at work, we were there together. I think those days were good for us both . . . and I know they are ones I will never forget.

The months moved along, and going to work each day became more difficult than ever for Don. In the past, he eagerly mixed with other employees. Now he withdrew unto himself, and spent more and more time working alone.

Emotionally, he was hurting.

Late in 1989, more than a year after the initial diagnosis, Don was informed that he was to be transferred from the technical spot in his engineering unit to the nearby training center where he had taught many classes during past years. The center had a surge of students coming in, and they needed some added expertise. Don was a highly-respected instructor, and when they requested help from his unit, his name was mentioned as a possibility. None of the men under whom he was currently working knew what to do about Don Miller, and perhaps for them the move seemed like a perfect solution.

The possibility that Don might be suffering from Alzheimer's disease was not something we were ready to admit to ourselves, much less disclose to others, and the group at the training center was unaware that he was having problems. They were delighted to have Don in their midst, and opened their minds and hearts to him. But gradually, that fine group of men and women began to discover that something was very wrong. Soon, compassion and empathy became mixed with the respect many of them held for the knowledgeable, dedicated, and caring man they had known over the years.

One of the last scenes from his year at the training center is vivid in my mind. Don was to teach a class on motors. During the evenings before the class, he spent long hours gathering material, trying to prepare. We had a finished basement area that was carpeted and paneled, where I had my typewriter and he had his desk and books. One evening I went down to see how he was doing.

Little piles of paper were spread all over the rug, and Don seemed perplexed and frustrated. As he responded rather eagerly to my query about the possibility of helping, I began to realize what kind of a jumble existed in his thoughts. He was trying to put in order, and assemble, probably 50 sheets of paper that he wanted to place in a notebook. He had made one copy of some pages, several copies of others, and had missed another group. With no technical background regarding motors, it all looked like "Greek" to me. I stood there feeling completely helpless.

Suddenly I noticed that he had an index listing sitting on his desk. I picked it up. Perhaps it would hold the keys to making order out of the chaos. Slowly and carefully we got piles in order, noted what was missing, made a list of what needed to be found and copied. The next morning I went over to the center with him. We copied the necessary sheets, and put them all together.

I knew we both hoped for a successful class, but when it came to presenting the material, I learned later that the situation rapidly became a disaster. This man who had given so many fascinating and stimulating classes on similar technical topics, who had helped clear the vision of so many engineers of all ages on the same subject many times in the past, simply could not do it that day. Fortunately, the coordinator of that group of students was sitting in on the presentation. That compassionate young engineer quietly and tactfully clarified and supplemented Don's efforts, and saved the day.

During the fall of 1990, the number of students at the training center returned to normal, and Don was transferred back to the technical unit. This move must have confused him even more. I could tell that he was just "putting in time."

In February of 1991, Don's current manager and the personnel man from the group asked for a meeting with Don and me at our home. All of us were well aware that Don's reasoning powers were limited at the time, but no one mentioned that fact.

After introductory pleasantries, his manager got right to the point. "How would you feel about taking 'early retirement' starting March 1, Don?"

It was absolutely silent for a few moments. Then slowly and hesitantly Don replied, "I guess that would be okay . . . "

Their request surprised me, and without even thinking, I blurted out my own response. "We have no financial plans in place for Don to retire so soon. I don't think we can afford to do that.

"He will be 62 in July," I continued as my thoughts raced ahead. "He would still not be eligible for the full pension or social security benefits that he would receive at age 65, but at least retiring at 62 would be better than doing so now, when he is only 61."

On impulse, I suggested a "lack-of-work" status, where he would receive his regular corporation paycheck for the next four months, even if he weren't working.

They said that was something they could not justify.

With more confidence than I felt, I quietly repeated, "We can't afford to have Don retire right now."

A stalemate.

The two men stayed a bit longer, we exchanged small talk, and they left.

What had possessed me, I wondered after they left. Why had my response been so adamant? I began to feel extremely insecure about the entire episode. But I wasn't nasty, I tried to reassure myself. I was just stating the facts of which I was well aware. We simply were not financially prepared for Don to retire early with partial benefits. We had not discussed or planned for such an event. It was not that our financial affairs were in such bad shape. They were not. Ever since Don had started with the company, we had carefully saved the maximum amount from his paycheck in the savings and security plan. We were frugal with our spending — frugal in our entire lifestyle — but we were not prepared to consider retirement on March 1!

Don had remained with one company for his entire career — unusual in today's business environment — with the conviction that being part of a large corporation provided some extra security. We were grateful for the savings plan, for the pension plan, for the medical coverage the company provided. However, under different circumstances Don would have worked until he was at least 65 — which would have given him three more years to enjoy his engineering work, three more years of full salary, a larger retirement package, and full social security benefits. I had enough money sense to know that in spite of our careful spending and saving habits, we would suffer long-term financial consequences if Don were forced to retire early.

I was astounded, when a few days later I was invited to the plant to participate in a second meeting with Don and those two men. They had a letter prepared. He was to leave his position on March 1, 1991. He would receive a lack-of-work status, with full pay and benefits until he reached age 62 in July. The letter stated that he had reviewed the opportunity with his wife, and that he was leaving voluntarily. The document was to be signed by him, and they requested that I add my signature. The status would never have been approved, the two men said, if it weren't for Don's many years of service with the company, and the outstanding reputation that he had built over those years. Although I do not think that Don was able to comprehend the complete meaning of what we were signing, or of the words being said, I was grateful for both.

As the two men spoke of Don's reputation, spoke about the respect others had for him, I thought about the last two and a half years when day after day he had gone to work, faced the competitive corporate world, tried to cope, with his confusion obviously worsening, and the diagnosis of Alzheimer's disease haunting him. My respect for him soared even higher.

In July, when it came to all the paperwork connected with retirement, I was the one who had to make every decision. As each option was presented, I realized that Don's careful choices all along the way had laid excellent ground work. It was my responsibility not to bungle it. As we sat together in a conference room on that hot summer day of 1991, with Don simply acquiescing to any comment or suggestion I made, I was deeply concerned about that burden.

One large decision was connected with what pension benefit option we should select for his retirement years. We could take a lump sum of the entire amount when he retired. Or we could take what they called the 50 percent option, where one received a calculated monthly sum immediately and for as long as the employee lived, but upon the employee's death the surviving spouse would get half of that sum each month. The third option was to take what they called the 100 percent option, where one would receive a lesser monthly check, but upon the employee's death, the surviving spouse would continue to receive the same monthly payment until his or her death.

I tried to wrap my mind around the choices. It was so complex . . . but it did seem to me that under the circumstances in which we found ourselves, the 100 percent option made great sense.

It was carefully presented to me that most people take the 50 percent option — the choice that allows them to maintain the larger monthly income as long as the retiree is living.

But, we weren't most people. Our situation was a bit different. A rather devastating diagnosis had been delivered. I had no idea what the future would hold, but I knew I had better consider the idea that Don was very likely to pre-decease me.

I insisted that we take the 100 percent option. I knew how to be frugal. I would find ways for us to live on the lesser monthly sum. And the company did provide good coverage that would help with whatever costs lay ahead as far as medical expenses.

We had to check one of three small boxes. I knew that was the box we should check, the alternative we should take.

Every time the first of the month rolls around, I am grateful I made that choice.

And thus began our "Golden Years" of retirement . . .

Chapter Five

March first arrived, as did the second, the third, the fourth, and each day thereafter. The reality began to sink in for Don. He had no office to go to, no job, no "title," no career. He had worked long and hard in college and throughout his years in the corporate world to learn and improve his expertise as an electrical engineer, and the sense of satisfaction and self worth it provided abruptly disappeared.

Now suddenly Don found himself spending his days at home, not fully comprehending the change, and not knowing what to do with his time. There were occasions when he would try so hard to be cheerful and helpful, but gradually he became more tense and withdrawn. He was obviously frustrated, depressed, and a deeper anger than I had ever seen expressed openly by him began to appear.

One morning in early March, we both awakened early. I opened my eyes to find Don lying on his stomach, with his face scrunched into his pillow. As I reached out to touch him, his anger erupted.

"They 'shit' on me, and they go on 'shining' and 'looking great!' I tried to do a good job! They dumped on me! I'm nothing. A no-good, worthless engineer without a mind!" The anger, bitterness, and hopelessness was almost overwhelming him, and threatened to overwhelm me as well. Similar outbursts became a very common occurrence during that spring and summer of 1991, and I had much to learn, as I struggled to help Don — to calm him, to divert him.

Don was the top 440 yard man on his college track team. After he left school he seldom competed, but logged many miles each week just because he loved to run. I encouraged him to continue. He was still slim and trim, in excellent physical condition, and his graceful running form was a familiar sight in our neighborhood. Through the sharing of his expertise and joy of running with both Lisa and our older daughter, Sandy, they, too, had become fine runners. When the girls were still living at home, the three of them had laid out all kinds of routes throughout our small community. Because Don seemed to remember the shorter routes, and always made it home again — often in a better mood and thinking a little more clearly than when he'd left — I felt comfortable about urging him to go out for a run when weather permitted.

Sometimes we would take a long walk or work in the yard together.

Sometimes we ran errands in the mall, walked from one end to the other, and stopped for something to eat.

In an attempt to give some sense of structure and purpose to his day, I urged Don to walk over to a nearby store to get a paper in the mornings. (As I transcribe my notes about those years, I now wonder about his trips to the store . . . about his running. What if he really had gone to that nearby river, as he originally threatened to do . . . ?)

When he returned from the store, he would sit down to read the paper — but after briefly perusing it, he would lay it down. I wasn't sure if he simply lost interest, or if his ability to comprehend written words was slipping. He would not sit in front of the television set alone, but what a lifesaver the VCR was. Many evenings we curled up next to one another to watch a movie, and for those brief periods of time when Don seemed relaxed, I was almost able to forget the frightening aspects of our own lives.

We moved into the summer months, and Don's confusion mounted. Gradually, his ability to comprehend who I was began to diminish, to fade in and out.

"Pat is gone part of the time," he said one day. "I'm glad you are here. Stay as long as you can."

I remember my deep sense of shock and absolute disbelief when my husband of 38 years first made that statement . . . and it was only the first of many to follow. He said it so matter-of-factly . . . looking straight at me. How could he not know who I was? I'd been right there, right beside him throughout the years . . . as we shared our lives, our home, our bed. How could this be? And, who did he think I was? I was never sure . . . How difficult it must have been for Don . . . and how heartbreaking it was for me.

One day he said, "These people in the house. I feel violated!" On another day, with deep sadness in his voice, he said, "Why are you taking my house away from me? I have no other place. I'll be out on the street." I tried reassuring him with words and hugs. "This is your house, Honey. I'm Pat. We are married — we have been together for 38 years. We have two wonderful daughters, Sandy and Lisa. They are in their own homes now. There is no one else here in the house but us. Just the two of us." Sometimes it would help, sometimes it would not.

A few days later when once again I tried to reassure him, he became angry. "I'm tired of being told that you are my wife," he said. "That's a stale idea. I've heard it before. And I object to having all of these people in and out of my house!"

"Who are they?" I asked, trying to measure my words carefully.

"I don't know!"

"Am I one of them?"

"Yes!!"

"But . . . I'm Pat . . . we are married . . ."

"You like to say that so you can gain control! I'm monogamous! I married Pat Harris!"

I cautiously tried showing him my Social Security card, our photo album, my driver's license . . . all to no avail. Slowly it began to register in my head. Such efforts were useless.

A little later that evening he came into our bedroom, furtively shut the door and said, "There's a young woman downstairs, half my age, who says she is married to me. She even has documents to prove it. She even got out our photo album!"

His sincere face reflected both anger and concern. I simply did not know what to say. Slowly the words came out. "That was me, Don . . ."

For what seemed like an eternity, he just stared at me. Then with the most heartbreaking look he said, "I'm losing my mind, aren't I?"

My heart and my arms reached out to pull the two of us together. I held him. I kissed him. I sat on the bed and gently urged him down beside me. I quietly reminded him of all that we had been doing to find out what was going on . . . struggling to find words . . . Yet in spite of his momentary apparent awareness of the magnitude of the whole problem with which we were dealing, there seemed to be little reaction or comprehension of what I was saying. I soon stopped talking, and simply held him close. Then I urged him to lie down, curled up beside him on the bed, and we fell asleep in one another's arms.

In the fall of 1991, a new doctor we were seeing agreed to try an antidepressant, and started Don on a low dose. After a few weeks, things seemed a little better for him . . . almost, as Don put it, as though the "fog" had lifted a bit. In spite of the fact that the clarity wasn't consistent, he became excited. And so did I! We spent more time talking — about his retirement, the diagnosis we had been given, our trip to the diagnostic clinic and those doctors' assessment that it was not Alzheimer's disease, about the girls, about our love, about our life together. The doctor slowly increased the antidepressant, but that clarity continued to come and go. I never knew what to expect. One night he abruptly got up from his chair in the living room and went upstairs. I quietly followed him. He went into our bedroom, took off his shoes and slacks, and got into bed. I decided I had best do the same. I took a quick shower, crawled into bed, and snuggled up next to him. He pulled away with a jerk.

I got up and went downstairs to the den, feeling hurt . . . and tired. I pulled out my guitar and quietly strummed away on a few familiar songs, trying to calm my ragged emotions.

Suddenly at the door appeared my kind and gentle husband, in a mood that was so completely out of character for him.

"That's too noisy!" he declared. He stood there for a moment, just glaring at me, then he turned around and stormed back up the stairs.

At first I just sat . . . stunned. Then, no longer able to contain my feelings, I gave in to the tears. Soon sobs racked my body. I felt like I was living a nightmare. How could all this be happening . . . I cried and cried, as all the emotions, pent up for so long, rose to the surface. Gradually, my sobs subsided, and once again, I just sat . . . feeling completely drained and exhausted. Finally, I tiptoed back upstairs and quietly slipped into one of the girls' rooms for the rest of the night.

I was always grateful for the times when Don was less confused and seemed to see things more clearly. But I slowly began to realize that when he didn't, insisting that he comprehend my view of reality appeared to upset and confuse him even more. Simply agreeing with him, and possibly trying to divert him, helped the most.

As I struggled to find ways to respond to Don's changing perceptions, I suddenly thought of Viktor Frankl's book, *Man's Search For Meaning*. When Dr. Frankl was in a German prison camp, he decided not to awaken a fellow prisoner who was obviously having a nightmare, realizing that the nightmare might be better than the "real" situation there in the camp.

Maybe, I thought to myself, that is a concept I need to consider in this situation . . .

One November evening, we were sitting in the living room. I was trying to read. Don was holding a *National Geographic* magazine, but he was just sitting, and very quiet. I began to sense that he was looking at me with great intensity, obviously thinking and pondering.

"Are you from California . . . ?" he finally questioned.

"Yes," I responded slowly.

"Is your name Pat . . . ?"

"Yes . . . "

His eyes began to light up . . . then his words burst forth. "I found you, I found you! I thought I had lost you!!"

He got up from his chair and almost stumbled towards me, with a radiant look of joy covering his face. "Things seem different! I thought I was lost! I felt so alone! No money, no place . . . "

I rose to meet him and the two of us met, truly found one another, there in the middle of our living room. We embraced and clung to each other, and tears rolled down both of our cheeks.

My heart ached in that moment of recognition and clarity, and how I longed to not only hold Don, but also to clutch him "there" in that instant of intimacy between us.

When we crawled into bed a little later, his eyes met mine, and with a quiet, happy look of recognition he said, "I love you very much."

But a few evenings later he was talking to Sandy on the telephone about the "individual" who was there in our house. "A nice person, if I'm going to be with someone . . . " he told her. He would often choke up if he spoke of "Pat" from "California" — unable to connect me with that "Pat."

One dark and rainy evening, we were eating dinner at the kitchen table. I began to realize that for quite some time he had been sitting in silence, just looking at me, with an unbelievably sad and lost expression on his face.

"What are you thinking?" I asked.

There was a long pause. Then slowly his words came out.

"About five years ago . . . Pat and I . . . used to be together," he said, with long pauses between each phrase. "We moved . . . from somewhere . . . don't know what happened to Pat . . . but . . . I've never quite forgotten her . . ."

His heartfelt words threatened to overwhelm me.

What to say . . .

I paused, struggling with my own emotions . . . searching for a response. I couldn't resist trying.

Looking deep into his eyes — seeking to reach the soul of that man of mine — slowly, carefully, I said, "Honey . . . it's me. I'm Pat . . . "

He looked at me, and shook his head ever so slightly.

"No . . . " he said slowly. "A different Pat. My Pat."

He simply could not see "me."

A deep, pervading sadness filled my being. In spite of efforts to control my emotions, tears began to roll down my cheeks. Don, too, was in tears. I knelt down beside him, and wrapped my arms around him. His arms enfolded me . . . and we held one another.

We were so close . . . yet so very far apart.

As the months wore on, I knew that I needed to do something more, to get help for both of us. Helping Don through the day, and keeping up with the multitude of things that required attention in our home and in our lives, was becoming increasingly difficult. And I was struggling with my own frustration and fear, as well as a building fatigue. I still did not want to acknowledge Alzheimer's disease, but there was no question in my mind that for Don, things were getting worse.

His frequent comments about heading for the river frightened me. Sometimes when he became upset. he would turn the anger in on himself and retreat into a deep depression. There were times when he would sit in the basement with the lights off, not wanting to talk, not wanting to eat, not wanting to do anything but sit.

I felt strongly that I needed to find someone else locally, who would not only look at Don's situation with knowledge, experience, and an open mind in regard to the diagnosis, but also who might consider conducting further tests. For my own peace of mind, I needed to get an opinion that could settle all the questions that, to me, still seemed unanswered. Was it denial? I can wonder, as I look back.

Perhaps. But I continue to feel that my questions were valid ones, and I know I didn't want to ever look back and have any doubts about having done all I could for Don.

I learned about a nearby psychiatric hospital with a fine reputation. Perhaps it was a place where I could find that someone. I spoke to Don's doctor about the possibility. He was open to the idea, and seemed to understand my feelings, my need to seek more information.

One cold and dreary day late in January 1992, Don was upset, and getting angrier by the moment. Nothing I tried seemed to help. I was almost at my wit's end, and completely worn out myself that morning. I called Don's doctor, and we agreed that I should contact the hospital to find out if they might be able to see Don that day, and possibly make some kind of assessment or recommendation. "Come," said the kind voice at the other end of the line when I called. "We'll have one of our psychiatrists talk with your husband, look at the situation, and see what we think."

I was slowly able to convince Don that we should see if we could find some help. He seemed just as tired and lost as I felt. I think we were both ready for almost any kind of action that might ease our situation. I packed a small bag for him, just in case they decided to admit him, and we headed for the hospital.

I was aware of the general location of Pine Ridge Hospital, but had never been there. I drove along the interstate, got off at the designated exit, and followed the directions I had been given. Before long, the sign I was looking for appeared. I pulled into the winding road that led toward a group of one-story buildings surrounded by well-kept grounds and tall pine trees. I parked the car in the visitor's lot, took Don's hand, and we walked toward the entrance.

Soon after our arrival, we found ourselves in a consultation room with a Dr. Stapleton and the male nurse assisting him. The warm and caring greeting we received almost overwhelmed my frayed emotions. Slowly, I began to relax, soon felt comfortable, and very aware that Dr. Stapleton was someone with whom I identified. His kind and carefully phrased questions were direct and perceptive, and he included both Don and me in the discussion. Although Don was not able to respond to most questions, and generally deferred to me, he, too, seemed more relaxed. It was almost with eagerness that he responded that, yes, he would like to have them see if they could help him.

Later that morning, after talking with us, studying the records I brought, and consulting with other members of the staff at the hospital, Dr. Stapleton met with us again, and suggested that we admit Don. They wanted to gather information over the next weeks. They would run some tests, include Don in a variety of group activities and therapy sessions, and work with him on a one-on-one basis.

"We will concentrate on pseudo-dementia and post-traumatic syndrome," he said. "We feel we may be able to help," he added, with a sincere and direct look.

As we left his office, his firm handshake spoke to me just as eloquently as his words. For the first time in many months, I felt a sense of peace. And how grateful I was for the medical coverage provided by the company for which Don had worked.

By noon, Don was settled in a semi-private room in one of the units. We had lunch together, took a walk, and I left to run a few errands at the nearby mall. I returned for dinner and spent the evening with him, hoping to help him adjust to the change. I began to realize that I, too, needed to adjust . . . to come to terms with the idea of actually leaving without him. How difficult it was to head for home that evening. I finally gathered my courage, assured him that I would be back the next day, gave him a hug and a kiss, and walked resolutely down the hall toward the exit.

As the big door to the unit swung shut behind me, I paused to look back through its windows. Don looked so lost, so alone, as he stood there watching me leave. My immediate impulse was to rush back in, take his hand, and hurry out the door together. I swallowed hard, and just stood for a moment. Then I smiled into those familiar blue eyes, blew him a kiss, and walked around the corner. I forced myself to walk to the car, get in, and drive home, alone, with tears streaming down my cheeks the entire way.

I visited Don every day while he was at Pine Ridge. The trip between our home and the hospital took about 45 minutes each way, and I usually played the radio or cassette tapes while I drove. Enya's *Watermark* repeatedly found its way into the tape deck, and those songs became hauntingly familiar. Often my vision became clouded with tears as I drove back and forth along that busy, fast-moving highway. The whole scene seemed so unreal in many ways, like a bad dream from which we might soon awaken.

But it wasn't a dream.

Dr. Stapleton shared that some of the tests they wanted to take included an EEG, and MRI, in order to compare them with those we had taken in the fall of 1988 with the local doctor, and in early 1989 at the diagnostic clinic. One morning, I drove to the hospital to take Don across town, where those images would be taken. On previous visits he had been fairly cheerful, but when I arrived that day, he was sitting on the bed, almost glassy-eyed, and obviously upset. Even though I was not sure he knew exactly who I was, his face reflected delight when I walked in the door of his room. But after a long embrace, all the fear that must have been building up, came rolling out in one heartbreaking sentence.

"I'm afraid I'm going to be a vegetable . . . "

I hugged him, tried to reassure him, told him I loved him very much . . .

But deep in my heart, I, too, was afraid.

I could work on coping with my fears, but Don did not have that capability. How frightening the whole scene must have been for him. He really didn't know where he was now. And when he was home, he didn't always recognize it as our home. It is difficult to imagine what it was really like for him to be living the nightmare. One factor I noticed in the weeks that Don was at Pine Ridge was that I seemed to have become his ally and a trusted friend, instead of one he sometimes viewed with suspicion or anger.

There were times when he wanted to talk to me, or at least "someone" at "home," on the telephone. He would become extremely frustrated with his inability to understand how to dial or use the telephone receiver. The nurses would dial the number for him when he asked, or when he was upset, and they felt that my voice could have a calming effect. Always, over those next years, Don seemed to recognize, and be comforted by, the sound of my voice on the telephone.

After he had been at the hospital for almost two weeks, we met with Dr. Stapleton and one of the hospital psychologists. We discussed the various tests they had taken, and how they compared with the results of the identical tests taken three years earlier. Their neurologist could see no changes in the EEG and MRI, not unusual even if they concurred with the Alzheimer's diagnosis. However, they shared that after analyzing all of the information they had, and observing and talking with Don for the two-week period, they continued to feel that they might be able to help him. They considered pseudo-dementia a real possibility! Their plan was to work with him, start him on a different antidepressant, gradually increase it, and treat his problems as severe depression. If those steps did not help, they would consider electric shock treatments (ECT).

ECT sounded like a frightening possibility to me, but the idea that we might actually be able to help Don was an unbelievably wonderful thought. What an awesome result to contemplate. I was afraid to hope. Their words were surely welcome ones, but a strong sense of caution pervaded my thoughts. "Wait and see. Take one day at a time," I kept repeating to myself.

I asked Dr. Stapleton if I could bring Don home for a weekend. He agreed to my suggestion.

How good it was to be together in our own house! We had a special dinner. I popped popcorn, and we watched a video that first night. What a treat to curl up together on our own couch in our cozy den. Did he know it was his home? I didn't know, but as the weekend progressed, I doubted that he did.

He watched carefully for cues from me in order to know what to do, and tried so sincerely to help in any way he could. As had been the case recently, there wasn't much conversation, but at dinner Saturday night, he began to struggle with words, trying so hard to express himself. He said he was afraid of dying . . . and with deep emotion reflected in his voice, face, and eyes, he attempted to share his feelings.

His emotion struck responding chords of fear that resonated throughout my entire being. In spite of my strong belief that death could not truly separate us, that we would somehow be together again one day, I was nevertheless unnerved by the idea of losing him physically.

Even though it was early, I suggested we go upstairs to bed. I helped him take a warm bath, took a quick one myself, and lay down beside him. The closeness of simply lying there next to one another seemed to bring a reassuring sense of security to us both that night.

Very little of the behavior that had been so difficult during the last months at home surfaced, but by Sunday afternoon, Don was restless. He told me he should be "getting back." Driving back along the same route I had taken just two days before, he said something about whoever had picked him up had gone way "West," taken a different road. Those years of struggling with that disease must have been so very confusing for him, perhaps something like driving along in a fog, where things fade in and out to the point that one cannot maintain an accurate sense of reality.

Dr. Stapleton and the doctors with whom he worked, gradually increased the dosage of the antidepressant, but the results were not what they had hoped. Finally, they suggested that we consider the ECT treatments. In response to my questions and concerns, Dr. Stapleton said he felt ECT was less dangerous than the potential side-effects from larger doses of the antidepressant. We agreed to try it.

After the first several treatments, there were some very positive effects, and we were all encouraged. Don and I would work in the evenings at remembering names of family, friends, past events . . . and his successes were exciting and fun for both of us.

One morning, I picked Don up and brought him home again, with the agreement that I would bring him back the following day. He cried, with what seemed to be tears of recognition, when we pulled up to the house. We had a wonderful time! We took a walk, and had lunch. I trimmed his hair. We took a shower together, took a nap, had dinner. Later, I built a fire in the fireplace and we listened to some favorite music, and talked . . . about the possibility of depression causing his problems, about our daughters, about my identity. Many times during the day and evening, he looked at me for a moment or two, and then said with great emotion, "I love you very much."

The next day, I met with Dr. Stapleton and the psychologist. They asked what I thought. I shared some of what I was seeing, finally shrugged my shoulders, and said, "I don't know what to think." They looked at one another and laughed, shrugged their shoulders, and said they didn't know what to think either, but that they saw a big change, and thought that Don seemed to have improved in many areas.

They said they were beginning to wonder if there really may have been a gradually building depression that set him on a downhill spin where he became almost psychotic. Their neurologist had questioned the idea of Don's problems being neurological, and they were seriously questioning the idea as well. Both said they were a bit excited, intrigued, and a little hopeful. They had Don come in to join our meeting, and he looked and sounded much better than he had in recent months.

A young engineer friend of Don's was in town and inquired about visiting. "Perhaps the three of us could meet for dinner at the Chinese restaurant that is close to the hospital," I suggested.

We agreed to meet the following evening, and how pleasant it was to find myself in a more "normal" setting. Don spent most of the time quietly listening, I enjoyed the casual, yet stimulating conversation with his friend, and I think all three of us enjoyed the special oriental dishes. Some people have difficulty relating to a person with problems similar to Don's, but this young man was kind, tactful, and understanding.

After dinner, I took Don back to Pine Ridge, stayed with him for awhile, then headed for home. It had been such a pleasant evening, reminiscent of so many dinners with friends in the past . . . "Could it be that it is truly just depression that we have been fighting?" I asked myself as I drove along the busy interstate. It was an awesome and exciting idea to contemplate! I had to work at reminding myself to restrain those building hopes.

And it turned out that our enthusiasm was short-lived. Don's more positive and hopeful attitude, and the times of seeming clarity, became more fleeting, and less frequent. After a total of six ECT treatments, the doctors at Pine Ridge decided to discontinue them. The medical team at the hospital had believed it was worth a try, and because of my great respect for the group, I had agreed. In retrospect, I am glad we tried it. Would I do it again? Yes. I would never leave any stone unturned.

By now I was well aware that doctors usually come to a diagnosis of Alzheimer's disease by the process of elimination. Considering all the circumstances in Don's life that had preceded the symptoms, it was important to me to find a way to rule out depression. Similar to the experience of the staff at the diagnostic clinic, this group's early studies led them, too, to think that the difficulties Don was experiencing might well be caused by something other than a neurological problem. But that was not to be the reality for us.

In early March of 1992, we checked Don out of the hospital with directions to continue on the antidepressant they prescribed, and appointments for regular visits with Dr. Stapleton.

Chapter Six

As we left Pine Ridge, one member of the medical team asked if I was ready to "place" Don. "Place him?" I answered that I didn't think so! Would she be if it were her husband!? "Perhaps not . . ." was her quiet reply.

My response to her question had been immediate and spontaneous, in spite of the fact that I was now very aware that I needed to acknowledge the diagnosis of "Probable" Alzheimer's disease. The idea of moving Don into a nursing home was heartbreaking . . . more than difficult to contemplate. I didn't even want to think about it.

How challenging it was to make decisions about and for Don. We had always valued our ability to think out loud with one another, to discuss the choices we made. For the past several years all decisions had been mine alone to make — and here was another question that required a decision, one that would deeply affect us both. The responsibility felt like an incredibly heavy one.

As I grappled with the nursing home question during the following months, I found myself struggling with old "tapes" from childhood, demands to follow certain "shoulds" — demands that as an adult I often tended to put on myself. I was aware that some of what was behind my not wanting to utilize a facility was the feeling that I should be "perfect" and should be able to take care of the man I loved in our own home.

Intellectually, I knew the quality of care and what I was comfortable with were the important factors, not where the care took place, nor what anyone else thought I should do. I knew there were no "right" answers, that there was no "right" way to cope. But nevertheless, it was still easy for my thoughts to become muddled, for my feelings to take over and make it difficult to think clearly.

If any disease is part of a loved one's life, it is part of our lives as well. How we deal with that reality becomes such an individual matter. I needed to find what was right for us, and not think that my choices needed to measure up to anyone else's ideas . . . and I needed to be careful about those "shoulds."

I sought inputs from family members, from special friends, from trusted people in the medical profession — but I knew that the actual decisions were mine alone to make. And as vulnerable as I felt at times, I knew I must remember that I did not need to defend my decisions.

A friend helped me log on to America Online (AOL) on her computer, and we discovered a "Senior Forum." There, we learned about an Alzheimer's chat room, and I felt most accomplished when I was able to follow her guidance and find my way to that site. I found a suggestion from one caregiver that really clicked. "Think of dementia this way, folks," the gentleman wrote. "The person you knew is silently standing beside this confused shell of themselves, and they are pleading with you to follow what they would have wished for you and themselves. Think of this whenever your self-control and self-confidence become shaky."

My self-confidence was shaky . . . but when I was first asked the question about utilizing a facility, I knew immediately that I was not ready to "place" Don. Would I be ready in the future? In reality, no. Never. Would I eventually have to be ready? I didn't know. I would try to take that one day at a time. I would talk to people, ask questions, seek inner guidance, follow my heart . . . and walk on.

I would find the way that was right for Don, for me . . . for us.

As the challenges at home mounted, there were times when I felt a strong sense of not being "alone," of being aware of that which I sense as God . . . a Power . . . a Presence that I knew in my heart was there to guide and sustain me. But in spite of my beliefs, it was difficult to stay "tuned in."

Often I was blindly trying to cope, and would forget to be open to any kind of inner guidance. I knew that it was not only vital that I stay "tuned," but equally important to work on my attitude. How I responded to each moment, each situation, was crucial, not only for me, but for both of us. My attitude, my responses, deeply affected Don's attitude and responses.

I drove Don to Dr. Stapleton's office for weekly appointments, and also scheduled times when I was able to talk with the psychiatrist myself. The atmosphere at Pine Ridge was an informal one, and Dr. Stapleton encouraged Don and me to call him David. I sensed a common spiritual bond with David, which helped me feel comfortable about discussing my thoughts and feelings, as well as my faith with him.

Being able to talk out loud about the situation was invaluable. I found that David's questions helped me find my own answers, and when I began to lose my perspective, I was very grateful for his.

One evening, a woman leading a support group I attended said to those of us seeking to learn from one another, that the scene would continue to get worse and worse — just what we needed to hear. Soon afterwards, I told David, almost in a panic, "It's going to get worse and worse!"

"No," he said quietly, "It will be different."

As soon as he said the words, I knew that he was right — and knew I had fallen back into "eating elephants . . . "

But even with David's help, it was difficult to keep my perspective — to keep my balance. I found it extremely challenging to find ways to keep Don busy, semi-happy, and safe. Bills poured in. Papers piled up. As I spent growing amounts of time meeting Don's needs, our home and all of our personal matters were becoming sorely neglected.

Both Sandy and Lisa were married, and they both lived in the South. We spoke on the telephone frequently and regularly, and they each came up several times a year. But they were not nearby to help. We had good friends who did live in the area, and they repeatedly reminded me that they were there for us. But I was well aware that they had challenges of their own with which to cope, and was careful about how often I took them up on their offers.

Finally, I heard the small voice in my head.

I had to find help.

I contacted our church, and the Stephen Ministry group asked one of their trained volunteers to see if he could assist in some way. Mike soon became a treasured friend. That big, gentle soul of a man, with his infectious grin, kind and under-standing heart, arrived at our door one evening. I eagerly accepted his offer to visit with Don while I went to a support group meeting or ran errands. He and Don got along famously, and soon Mike and I got along famously as well. From the moment Mike arrived on the scene, he was there whenever and wherever we needed him. What would we have done without Mike?

Or without Frank, a long-time engineering friend from Don's corporate unit. Frank was a fine technical person and a warm-hearted, sensitive man. Every so often this loyal friend would take Don to lunch, to company functions, or for walks by the river. Sometimes he simply visited, but Frank, too, was always there for Don.

Seeking more aid on a daily basis, I talked with members of the support group, people at the Office for the Aging, other health-related agencies, and many people in our community about what help was available. I tried utilizing both men and women from home-care related employment agencies, tried taking Don to a senior lunch and activity site at a neighborhood church, and accepted the offer of regular visits from a friend who was a private-duty Registered Nurse (R.N.). Although some of these efforts worked well, some did not, or soon became inadequate. I began having Don spend part of each day at the Senior Citizen's Centercare facility.

In our original interview, the woman in charge suggested that I should not wait too long before we used a full-time facility. She commented that younger people with Alzheimer's often move through the various stages of the disease more quickly than older people, and quietly added that because of current laws in our state, it might be wise to look for a place that had both an adult home and a nursing home unit. A person could only remain in an adult home as long as he or she was continent. When that control was lost, it was necessary to move to a nursing home. She shared that nursing home beds were scarce, and being accepted into a facility's adult home usually provided "priority access" into their nursing home section.

Again, the suggestion of utilizing a nursing home. And incontinent . . . Yes, I realized, there were some incidents that made me wonder if we were moving in that direction more rapidly than I had thought we might. Several times I had found Don washing out his underpants, obviously embarrassed as he told me that he "just hadn't gotten there . . . "

For a while using Centercare seemed to work well for Don, and how I appreciated the break it provided for me. Their bus would stop for him in the mornings, and I would pick him up each afternoon. On the way home in the car, he would often say something about being at work, and discuss the "job." The idea that he had a place to go during the day that seemed like "going to work" appeared to be helpful for him.

But those next months were filled with the now familiar contrasts. There were many days when Don was smiling and cheerful about going to Centercare, but also times when he expressed anger about going back to "that place!" When he was upset about going, it was easy to feel guilty about utilizing their help. I would have to remind myself that his perception, his attitude toward something, could flip very quickly even when he was home.

Many times Don's frustration, sadness, and depression threatened to engulf me. David suggested that I remember that Don's attention span was short, that he would forget quickly, and to use that to our advantage. He suggested that I try to change a scene by moving on and distracting Don, as well as myself, rather than letting us both get caught in his illusions, in his blackness.

I began to notice that on many occasions Don became extra confused or agitated in the evenings — a phenomenon I later learned is often experienced with Alzheimer's disease and referred to as "sundowning." I tried reading some of our favorite poetry to him as we sat together in front of the fire, often with tapes playing softly in the background. It seemed as though the physical closeness, the sound of my voice, and the quiet music were calming influences.

One night, the words of a Roger Whittaker tape suddenly began to register in my thoughts.

"Hold my hand, and we'll fly away."

Oh, how I wished we could . . .

There was a meeting at Centercare one evening when Mike was not available. I decided to go anyway, and to take Don with me. I asked him if he would wait for me in the lounge, took some magazines for him to look at, left the door ajar, and kept a careful eye out through the room's large window to make sure he was still there.

When we finished our meeting, I walked out to where he was sitting. We exchanged grins as I approached, and I thanked him for waiting for me. He looked me in the eye as I reached for his hand, and then he said, "I'd wait anywhere for you."

The sincerity of his words, the love in his eyes, the warm clasp of the familiar hand that reached for mine, made my heart soar. It didn't matter that I wasn't sure if he knew who I really was. I knew who he was. I loved him. And I knew he loved me.

As I lay in bed that night, I thought about the fact that last fall I'd been trying to help Don know that he was in his own home, that I was his wife. This fall, I was just trying to let him know that I loved him, that he was safe, and to make life as simple and as pleasant as I could. Working on not trying to pull him back to what I perceived as reality definitely seemed to be helpful for us both, and I was grateful for the times when his love for me, or at least his loving nature, burst forth, as it had that evening.

Often, I simply could not get to sleep at night. Don's unconscious movements, and occasional talking or mumbling, made it difficult. There were many times when I drifted off, found myself awakened, and in frustration quietly slipped out of our bed and moved to one of the girls' rooms. But if Don awoke and found me gone, he seemed to feel that the lack of my presence meant it was time for him to get up. Many times I would groggily "come to," and realize he was up and moving around the house in the middle of the night.

Mike helped me move one daughter's twin beds into our room. We pushed them together and I made them up as one, hoping that would help keep me from being disturbed by Don's movements. I arranged to have deadbolts placed on the front and back doors, and locked them at night so if Don did get up he couldn't just wander outside. (Perhaps not a good idea in case of fire, I realize in retrospect.) But still I was not comfortable if he began wandering around inside the house at night. In spite of the various things I tried, lack of sleep remained a problem and began to take its toll on me.

I was tired. The break that the hours at Centercare provided was becoming increasingly vital. Often when I tried to catch up on paperwork during the hours that Don was at the center, I found I couldn't concentrate or keep my eyes open, and ended up asleep on the couch. On several occasions, I found myself feeling dizzy and almost disoriented as I drove along the interstate on my way to see David. And my weight was down ten pounds. I didn't mind losing a pound or two, but I was well aware that this might not be the best way to be doing it.

After we had been utilizing Centercare for several months, I received a call from the woman in charge of the program. There were more occasions when Don was upset or angry. They were having trouble finding ways to calm or divert him, and his actions were upsetting to others in the group. She understood my reservations about using a nursing home, but I really needed to find one very soon, she concluded, and suggested several possibilities.

I was having a hard time dealing with the feelings of loss, the feelings of guilt, that plagued me when I utilized Centercare part of each day. How on earth would I ever deal with using a full-time facility? I didn't know.

As David watched me struggle with our daily challenges, he occasionally mentioned the idea of my using an antidepressant. Not pushing, simply holding out the idea as a possibility. A good way to approach a person who thought she "ought" to be in control, and not need that kind of support. It was there, if I needed it. I could decide. That fall, I knew it was time. I began taking a low dose of Zoloft.

I decided to try a special night out for the two of us, and made reservations to see a visiting Russian Chorus and Dance Ensemble one Saturday evening. Throughout the day, I kept reminding Don that we had a "date" that night. He was in a decent mood all day, and the evening went fairly well. But when we got back from the concert, he became confused. He couldn't figure out what to do with his coat, and apologetically tried to say that he was new there, that he wasn't too familiar with things. Then he became upset, saying he had no money. I assured him that it was okay, that there was plenty of money for us both. Next, he asked how far I had to go for the night. He seemed to know my first name, but obviously not my relationship to him.

I encouraged him to come upstairs with me, and filled the tub with warm water for a bath for him. He got in, washed, got out, and dried off. Then he became quite insistent about repeating the whole process. Along with the extra confusion, he was struggling to keep his balance. It was difficult to help him get into pajamas and ready for bed. He became increasingly upset, and soon I was close to tears. What I thought might be a pleasant diversion, a night out, a "date," had only served to confuse him more.

Suddenly I knew. I had to work at flipping the scene. A hug, an understanding comment, a small joke about our struggles, soon made all the difference. How rewarding it was to see him slowly respond, to see a smile begin to form, as I finally got him settled into bed. I crawled onto the bed too, curled up next to him and gave him a hug. I kissed his face, kissed his neck, told him he was a very special person. For a while we just lay there together. Gradually, he fell asleep — with that grin still reflected on his face.

As I lay there beside him, I was suddenly engulfed with fatigue and emotion. Slowly my eyes filled, and tears began to roll down my cheeks. I was filled with an overwhelming mixture of love and respect for Don, and deep sadness for us both. As I struggled to control my emotions, I felt that familiar hand begin to pat my arm. I looked over at his face. His eyes were still closed. He appeared to be sound asleep. That half-grin still lingered. And he continued to gently pat my arm.

The Thanksgiving holiday, 1992, proved to be a turning point in my thinking. I ordered a "take-out" meal of chicken and dressing, potatoes and gravy, and mixed vegetables from Boston Market. I purchased a frozen pumpkin pie from the supermarket for dessert. When I began to set things out for dinner, Don seemed to be feeling very useless. I asked him to put the dressing in a bowl . . . and he carefully placed the whole container in the bowl I set out. I asked him to get the napkins from the pantry. He brought out the Cling Wrap box. He set his multi-vitamin pill on his plate and tried to pick it up with his fork. When we got to dessert, he picked up his whole piece of pumpkin pie with his fingers, and ate it bite by bite. I watched with a deep sadness, as we worked our way through that "Thanksgiving" day.

Centercare was closed for four days. The weather was cold and rainy, and those next days seemed to stretch out in an endless fashion. The VCR became our magic carpet. I rented a stack of videos, encouraged Don to curl up next to me on the couch, and with the flip of a button we were transported into wholly different worlds — worlds completely devoid of Alzheimer's disease.

We made it through the four-day holiday, but it took a huge toll on me. I felt completely drained, and was unbelievably grateful when Don greeted Centercare's driver quite cheerfully on Monday morning.

Our minister was a man with whom I felt very comfortable, and soon after Thanksgiving, I made an appointment to talk with him about our situation. In a kind and caring manner, he suggested that Don had needs that I could not meet at home, needs that Centercare was unable to meet, and that perhaps it was time for me to consider the next step.

When I talked with Sandy and Lisa, I shared some of the recent changes in their dad, and the comments and suggestions from the Centercare administrator and our minister. I knew they both felt badly about living so far away and not being able to help out. They were careful not to tell me what to do, but I could tell there was no question in their minds that we needed to make a change. When I said I simply wasn't sure Don was ready, or that I was ready, for that "next" step, Lisa tactfully and cautiously commented that no adult home or nursing home would take Don, if he were not appropriate for such a place. I knew she was speaking from her own experiences as an O.T. in the field . . . yet . . . Then one afternoon when I went to see David my thoughts and feelings came rolling out in a string of words — a rather common occurrence . . .

"Everyone I talk with seems to feel it is time for me to utilize some kind of facility on a full-time basis, some kind of more permanent setup for Don, and first their comments almost anger me, then they frighten me, then I can become defensive, then filled with guilt when I try to seriously consider the idea. In my head I'm not truly convinced that he is really at the point where I need to make that change, but in my heart I know the need may be a reality, yet I can feel so awful, so disloyal, about actually considering it. Then I think about the frustrations we both are experiencing, and the nagging fatigue that hounds me every day as I work at keeping him home, and . . . but I don't want to fail Don . . . I love him so very much . . ."

David listened patiently, and carefully. When I finally stopped to catch my breath, his response was a quiet one.

"I think he is there."

As I drove home that afternoon, all the recent inputs from caring people went around and around in my head. And there was that inner sense of guidance, that inner "knowing," that spoke to me equally clearly.

In spite of my reluctance to take that next step, I knew David's simple comment, "I think he is there," needed to be heeded.

Chapter Seven

I was struggling with my own health — Sandy, Lisa, David, Mike, and our minister were all encouraging me to utilize some kind of facility on a more permanent basis — and I really did know that I had no other option. During the hours that Don was at Centercare, I began my search.

Lisa shared some of the things she had learned working as a therapist in nursing homes. She talked with other occupational therapists, and with her husband, Bob, who worked in a health-related field. Together, we began to make a list of questions and requirements. As I went from place to place, looking at all types of facilities, I gradually learned what was available, and more about the environment I hoped to find. I expanded our list, and methodically documented information about, and my reactions to, each place I visited.

One was new and nice, but seemed too sterile and "hospital-like," too big and impersonal. Another one was smaller, but way out in the country. It gave me a confined feeling, a deep sense of people being isolated, left behind to die, that I found difficult to shake even after I left the facility. There was one administrator with whom I did not seem to relate well, which I sensed as a warning sign. In another facility, many residents were just parked in a wheelchair in the hallway, often isolated from one another, and appearing to be neglected. Some nursing homes had a distinct odor of urine, which bothered me . . .

If we were really going to use a facility of some kind, I finally decided that the only place with which I could feel comfortable was one called Wentworth. It was located about 20 minutes from our home. Although it was not strictly set up for Alzheimer's patients, their brochures, and the administrator with whom I spoke, stated that their staff was trained and experienced in helping residents with the disease.

I visited several times. Mike went with me to check it out. Lisa, Bob, and Sandy flew up to help appraise Wentworth. We all came away impressed, and everyone with whom I talked spoke with high regard for the facility.

The first time I drove up the long, winding driveway that led away from the busy road, I was delighted to find myself in a quiet, peaceful, wooded area. Wentworth was adjacent to a well-kept private golf course, and many majestic-looking trees added to the beauty of the picturesque setting. The main entrance was in a stately-looking, sparkling white building with dark-green shutters — a newer section of the structure ambled off to the left and another to the right.

Railings surrounded the wide front porch at the center of the building. Comfortable-looking benches and rocking chairs seemed to beckon. The front doors led into a lounge/lobby that was spacious and elegantly decorated. That room, as well as the equally attractive dining room across the hall, looked comfortable and inviting. Down the hall there was a small gift shop, and a paneled, well-stocked library.

There seemed to be corridors leading in all directions. One corridor led to a group of spacious apartments in the wing on the left. It was glassed-in, giving residents easy access to the lounge, library, and dining room in inclement weather, and a refreshing view of the outdoors as they walked back and forth. A hallway led to the nursing home area, and another glass corridor to the right led to the adult home section. I learned that residents were invited to bring some of their own belongings, giving the rooms a personal and cheerful appearance. Each time we walked through the nursing home area, I noted with satisfaction that it did not have an odor. Scattered throughout the facility there were cozy little nooks with comfortable furniture where people could gather. There were places to fix a cup of coffee or tea and a snack. It was a good-sized facility, but in spite of its size, the entire place had a warm, "homelike" atmosphere.

The activity room was a busy and fascinating-looking place, and Lisa was highly impressed with the occupational therapy department. An alarm system alerted the staff if a nursing-home resident wearing an ankle bracelet went out any of the main doors. Since wandering was a definite possibility for a person with dementia of any kind, that feature definitely was an important asset.

As the woman at Centercare had said might be the case, if one was admitted to Wentworth's adult home, one had "priority access" to their nursing home. That would eliminate the need to make a change to a completely new facility later, when Don needed more care than the adult home arrangement could provide. I liked that idea. And there was a hospital located ten or fifteen minutes away, I noted, as I carefully checked things off on my list of requirements.

All of us felt that if we needed to utilize a facility of some kind, Wentworth appeared to be an excellent choice. Even though I continued to struggle with my emotions about the decision, in early December, I applied for Don's admission.

I was definitely impressed with Wentworth. The only problem was the fact that the wait for admittance into their adult home could be as long as six months. The mental and physical exhaustion that I had sensed after the Thanksgiving holiday was continuing to plague me, and six months sounded like an eternity.

The idea of utilizing a facility during the week, and having Don home on weekends, began to develop in my mind. I had heard of various kinds of respite programs, and wondered if I could find a place to use on a temporary, "part-time" basis until there was an opening at Wentworth.

None of the larger adult home facilities would accept someone for a short-term, part-time stay, but I finally found a smaller, attractive adult home where the administrator, who was also an R.N., was open to the idea. Even more important, she felt they would be able to work with, and help Don.

The cozy-looking little white house was only a few miles from our home, and the friendly sign perched in front declared that it was called Sunnybrook. The administrator was a candid, sensitive woman, and our conversation was congenial and productive. We talked about Don, about our situation, and about the problems we were experiencing with the daycare situation. We both felt it might work well to utilize their help until Don could be admitted to Wentworth.

The place was clean and cheerful looking. The small staff appeared to be good-natured and warmhearted. The 16 residents seemed "upbeat," friendly, and well-cared for. As impressed as I was with Wentworth, I liked the intimacy of this smaller facility. I found myself wishing it was a nursing home facility as well as an adult home — that this arrangement did not have to be an interim situation.

It was difficult to make such important decisions that would deeply affect Don, even though I knew I had no other choice. Although the unusual suspicion about me that he had reflected when he first retired had never appeared again, it had unnerved me. I was grateful that we seemed to have passed that phase, and that he once again reflected the intrinsic trust he had always had in me. It was a trust I did not want to betray.

I knew I shouldn't just spring a change on him, and watched for appropriate opportunities and ways to share the idea of using Sunnybrook. His anger and frustration about being at Centercare did seem to be increasing . . . I knew he continued to connect his time there with a "work" situation, and that he was very ready to make a "transfer" . . . I alluded to that idea, a little vaguely, hoping it might help us ease into the new setup.

One day in mid-December, the two of us went over to Sunnybrook for lunch and part of the afternoon. A cheerful young woman named Joanne took Don under her wing. She quickly got him talking about his love of running, told him that she had been trying to do some running each day to get in shape, and suggested they run together in the afternoons. Don seemed enthusiastic about the running, and open to making the "job" change. A good beginning.

I decided to make arrangements to have him start at Sunnybrook the first week in January.

I wanted Don's room to look as much like home as possible, and to be a place that might feel like his own space. I planned to have him use his dresser from home, and purchased a new La-Z-Boy recliner, just like the ones in our living room. I bought a pretty antique-white single bedspread for his bed, similar to the one on our bed. I set out our small TV/VCR, as well as our portable radio/cassette player and some of his favorite tapes to take to Sunnybrook. I had enlarged and framed a picture that he had taken of a sweeping view of the sun setting across the unusually still waters of the lake we'd stayed at in 1989.

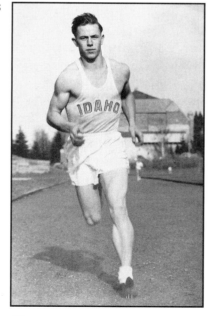

I remembered a large poster-picture of him running during his senior year in college. "That might be a fun thing to have in his room," I thought. When I retrieved it from the back of a closet, I was filled with memories of the pride I felt when I first spotted that 14" x 20" picture of Don Miller displayed in a drugstore window in the little town of Moscow before an important track meet! Proud that he was such a fine runner — and that I was his girl and he was my special guy! An 8" x 10" copy was soon framed and ready.

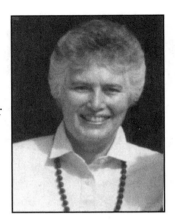

In a larger frame, I mounted a jaunty picture of Don standing in our front yard with his hands on his hips and a huge grin on his face, one of Sandy racing in a big college meet, and pictures of Lisa competing in a triathalon. I found a fairly new picture of me that could sit on his night stand.

With Don's appearance, behavior, and speech obviously deteriorating, I felt strongly that it was vitally important that anyone trying to help him should know more about who he was. It is so easy for any of us to judge a person by what we see with our eyes and hear with our ears. In order to give the staff extra guidance, I made a copy for their files of the information about Don's background that I had labored over for the diagnostic clinic. I included some updates about the current situation, added a note about the fact that he liked being busy and involved, and suggested that if they could find any simple tasks with which he might help, I felt sure he would respond positively. I carefully included copies of his living will and health care proxy form for their files.

I purchased a scrapbook and entitled it "Don's Book." I filled it with snapshots and printed comments in large letters below each picture, thinking that Don might look at it, and that whoever was helping him might look at it with him, or on his or her own. Even if Don did not recognize the scenes, I hoped the pictures might jog his memory, or warm his heart a bit. And perhaps they would help others engage him in a conversation, as well as know and understand him better.

When Mike came over for one of his regular visits with Don, I quietly shared my plans. He offered to help, and ended up taking everything over in his van, moving the furniture in, hanging the pictures, and setting up the room. He did a wonderful job. I was so very grateful for his help, for his special friendship, and for the trusting relationship he had been able to build with Don.

As I lay next to Don the Sunday night before we made that move, I thought about all my efforts to make the transition as smooth as possible for him. I was very aware that it would be a dramatic, and possibly traumatic, change for both of us. While he was at Pine Ridge, I knew that it was only temporary — knew he would be coming home again. This was different. He would probably never again be home on a permanent basis.

I wondered how Don would react to the change, how he would cope. And I wondered how I would react, how I would cope . . .

And so it was that in January of 1993, we began a new chapter in our lives. I planned to take Don over to Sunnybrook on Sunday nights, go for fairly extended visits several times during the week, and pick him up on Friday afternoons so we could spend our weekends at home together.

During the first week, the R.N. approached me quietly, suggesting that if I went ahead with that idea, I would see upsetting behaviors. I knew she meant well, but those behaviors were ones I had been seeing and dealing with for many months, and bringing him home for weekends was important to me. At the time, I felt that it would be helpful for both of us in making this transition. However, in retrospect I am not sure whether it was helpful, or confusing, to Don. At least my presence was always a constant, wherever he was, and there is no question in my mind that that remained important to him. And perhaps those weekends with him at home did help me gain some perspective, did help me truly comprehend with my whole being that Don really was leaving me — day by day, inch by inch.

I spent a fair amount of time at Sunnybrook during the weekdays. I could see how hard everyone worked at making Don feel welcome and comfortable. I felt equally comfortable, and the residents and staff soon began to seem like an extended family.

Don and Joanne tried running most afternoons during the week. Those outings were surely a different caliber of running from what he had done in the past, but the two of them seemed to thoroughly enjoy the fresh air and their trips up and down the road behind Sunnybrook. I am sure that the companionship and kindness Joanne showed Don meant a great deal to him.

With more time by myself, I often "thought out loud" on the typewriter. "Don't get isolated," I typed. "When you are depressed, reach out to others — they may be struggling with something, too. Call people when you are hurting. How can others help if they don't know what's going on? A few people seem to have pulled away. I think they may be frightened by Alzheimer's disease. I can understand. The disease has always frightened me. Scary to think one might have to walk this road . . . Scary to walk it . . .

"Over the years, I have often been afraid. But as I think about it, those fears were often connected with what-ifs about things that might lie in the future. This isn't the future. This is now. I have to walk this road. Some people have said, 'I couldn't do what you are doing.' I would have said exactly the same thing to them. Funny, when I come right up against something, and have to deal, I deal. It seems to me that is probably true for most of us.

"But I do have to keep concentrating on taking one step, one moment at a time, on not allowing myself to get overwhelmed by the big picture . . . and all the things that inevitably lie ahead.

"That 'elephant' does frighten me . . . but remembering the twinkle in Don's eyes when he showed me his simple sketch does help! Sometimes I feel guilty about his being at Sunnybrook during the week, and sometimes I feel okay about it. Then I feel guilty about not feeling guilty. Good grief, I know I could not have continued caring for him at home by myself on a full-time basis any longer."

Around and around my thoughts went, as my fingers flew quickly to keep up with my head. Often, just typing those ideas out and reading them later was valuable for clearing my thinking and gaining perspective.

When I called Sunnybrook one day, Joanne told me that some of Don's confusion disappeared when they went running. They shared jokes, talked back and forth, and his conversational skills seemed to improve. But when they got back inside, that clarity would disappear.

As she talked, I suddenly remembered something. When Don was still at home, there were times when he was angry or confused, and went out for a run. On many occasions, there would be a brief period after he returned when he appeared to be thinking a little more clearly, and often recognized me. It made me think, too, about the fact that he always was able to find his way home, at a time when there was a great deal of confusion in his mind about so many things.

Did that temporary change have something to do with oxygen? With endorphins? What was behind the phenomenon we observed? I still wonder today.

I continued my visits with David. One afternoon when we were talking, he made the comment that he felt at death, Don would be free. "Maybe you will be too," he added thoughtfully.

"Perhaps," I responded, "but I really feel almost guilty when I get a bit hopeful about a future for me, about possibilities for me later." With great empathy, David simply responded, "survivor's guilt," knowing I would understand just what he meant.

On another occasion, I was struggling with all kinds of negative emotions. Some of them were connected with the necessity to cope with all of the paperwork that kept piling up. There were papers connected with medical insurance, legal matters, and financial affairs. There were letters to be answered, forms to fill out, notices to respond to. There was a stack of bills to be paid . . . and a checkbook that needed to be balanced. And all of it needed to be attended to — by me.

"I can't do this!" I said in frustration.

"But you are," was his simple response.

I guessed that I was, but there were times when I felt completely over-whelmed, angry at the whole scene, sometimes abused, and definitely tired. I would often awaken struggling with depression. I sometimes had to almost make myself get up and get going in the morning, but as the day progressed, my mood would gradually change to a little more positive one. I was still taking a small amount of Zoloft. I had considered cutting it out completely, and it was at those times that I decided I was glad I had not done so.

Early in March, I received a call from the R.N. in charge of the adult home at Wentworth. They had a semi-private room available earlier than they had expected. (Don and I had visited their facility a few weeks before, wandered around a bit, met some people, and had lunch. I was well aware that he might not remember, but I had tried to set the stage for an upcoming change.) I thanked her for her call and told her we would like to utilize their room starting the next Monday, March 15.

Mike agreed to move Don's belongings from Sunnybrook to Wentworth while Don was home with me that next weekend. I knew he would do a good job of setting the chair in place, putting the pictures on the wall, setting everything up so that Don might be able to sense the familiarity.

When we arrived at Wentworth, I discovered that once again, Mike had done a wonderful job. We walked through the glass corridor, down the hall, and into Don's room — and there it was, looking almost exactly as it had at Sunnybrook. It had the added feature of a wide picture window, through which one could see a beautiful large maple tree in the center of a lovely snow-covered courtyard.

Don's roommate greeted us, but promptly went back to his television show. I was grateful for the curtain partitions, which allowed us some privacy.

I stayed with Don most of the day. The R.N. in charge of the unit took time to talk with us, introduce us to staff members and residents, and show us around. Later Don and I went exploring on our own. We talked with other residents, aides, the people in the activity room, and a delightful young woman at the reception desk. We had a nice luncheon and went back to his room to take a "nap." I found that afternoon time a welcome respite, as I dealt with the challenges of our lives during those years. Sometimes when we curled up on his bed together, Don slept. Usually I did not, but I am sure we both enjoyed the closeness the time alone together provided. That night I lay down beside him on the narrow hospital bed, and stayed until I was certain that he was sound asleep.

I brought all of our accumulated paperwork with us when Don moved to Wentworth — medical records, medications and dosage directions, Don's living will and health care proxy information, and all of my notes to help people know more about him. In spite of my availability and all of the information in his file, we had problems four days later.

On the evening of March 19, I received a call. The staff at Wentworth was sending Don to Brentwood Hospital's Emergency Room (E.R.).

I drove to the hospital as quickly as traffic permitted, and was soon walking down the hall of the emergency room, scanning each cubicle. No Don. I turned around to retrace my steps. When I spotted him on my way back through, it was easy to see why I had walked right by him.

He was lying on a gurney covered with a white hospital blanket. His eyes were closed, and his face looked gray. His usually well-combed hair was in disarray, and his glasses were missing. His appearance had been changing gradually, but I was used to seeing him in different surroundings and in a different state. He had, at first glance, just looked like someone I didn't know — an elderly gentleman waiting for help, there in the E.R.

For a moment I just stood there looking at him, surprised at his appearance, and the fact that I had walked right past him. Then I moved in to touch his hand and smile into the eyes that met mine.

Don gripped my hand, obviously glad to see a familiar face amidst the unfamiliar surroundings. I soon learned that he had been having difficulties with coordination and balance. During dinner, he had struggled to get his fork to his mouth to feed himself. He was unable to keep his balance as he stood or tried to walk, and later had trouble even trying to keep from tipping over as he sat on the bed.

The doctors examined him, did a blood workup. After several hours at the hospital, they still were not sure what had caused his problems. He seemed a little better, and they decided to send him back to Wentworth. We arrived back in his room, I got him settled in bed, and at last headed for home.

When I got to Wentworth late the next morning, Don was sleeping, but as soon as I got him up, I could tell things were definitely not "right." His balance was terrible, and he could hardly move his feet to walk.

I hurried to the nurses' station.

"Something is still very wrong . . . Don can't walk. He can't even stand up without losing his balance."

And, back we went to the emergency room.

This time, the doctor on duty decided that he was over-medicated! In spite of all of our efforts to make the transition from Sunnybrook to Wentworth a smooth one, the dosages of the medications Don was taking had obviously gotten mixed up, or somehow misunderstood.

All of a sudden my concern about what could be wrong turned to exasperation. I had moved Don to the very finest facility that I could find, and, after only four days, we had been to the hospital emergency room twice!

A few phone calls and conferences between all parties concerned, gradually straightened the medication out, and we headed back to Wentworth once again. I stayed with Don the rest of the day, all evening, and finally left after he fell asleep that night. I arrived at home a little after 11:00 p.m. — feeling almost ready for a trip to that E.R. myself.

Another problem connected with my struggles during those difficult times involved my hair. There definitely seem to be periods when my mental state can be measured by its length! Ever since college days, when money was scarce, I have usually cut it myself. It has a bit of wave and is not hard to manage, if it's not too short. Sometimes during those months and years when Don was sick, especially when my frustration level was high, I would grab my scissors, thinking I would just "fix" a spot here or there. As my frustration level rose, my "fixing" became more frequent — and my hair was getting a bit short.

When I got home from the emergency room that night, I took a shower and washed my hair. As I was drying and curling it, I peered into the mirror and spotted several areas that definitely looked a bit uneven! It was already shorter than I really wanted it to be . . . but on impulse, I grabbed my scissors. Maybe if I worked just a little on this spot, and that spot, it would look better . . .

But it didn't look better, and I knew it.

A few days later, I had lunch with a long-time friend. In a warm and sensitive manner, that very special woman tactfully said my hair looked very nice, and carefully added that with such a short cut, I might want to consider getting my ears pierced.

Ah, yes. A good idea. Can't fix my hair. Can't hibernate. Perhaps earrings would help.

The next afternoon, I went to the mall to get my ears pierced, an action both of our daughters had taken in their teens . . . The little pearl posts did look rather nice, and definitely helped take my eyes away from what hair was left!

Perhaps that small personal climax served a purpose! It surely got my attention, helped me laugh at myself, and may well have helped me keep my perspective in regard to the overwhelming scene with which I was faced on a daily basis.

During his first four days at Wentworth, Don had made two trips to the hospital emergency room — not the best beginning for his stay in an extended-care facility. But now the medications appeared to be in balance, his equilibrium and coordination seemed better, and I caught my breath.

I visited every day, spending part of the afternoon and evenings with him. I wanted people there to know more about Don, and felt that perhaps my frequent presence, the fact that I obviously cared about him, might help them provide him with better care. I wanted to let him know that my presence in his life was still a constant. And, I just wanted to be with him.

Several times I arrived and found him not looking as well-groomed as he had at Sunnybrook. One day his hair was uncombed and greasy. He wasn't shaved. I noticed a strong body odor and his slacks showed signs of being wet. I talked with the R.N. who was in charge of the adult unit. She was pleasant and seemed concerned about my frustrations. She would have the aides give Don a daily shower and keep a closer eye on his personal hygiene.

I soon discovered that it seemed to be difficult for the aides to find time to follow through on that request. As I got to know some of those friendly and pleasant women, I could see how very busy they were. I inquired about the procedure and protocol in regard to giving Don a shower myself. They had no objections, graciously helped me find towels, showed me the routine, and checked to see how we were making out. Whenever we emerged from the shower, my clothes were mighty wet, but Don looked neat, clean, and smelled like soap and shampoo. After he was dressed, he would cheerfully return greetings from the staff and residents, as we made our way up and down the halls and corridors.

Each weekend while he was at Sunnybrook, I brought Don home. Would it work again? Or, would doing so just make the whole transition more difficult? It was so hard to know for sure. I decided I wanted to try. Two weeks after his admittance to Wentworth, I brought him home for the weekend.

The next two days did not turn out as well as I had hoped they would. We struggled with his bathing and dressing. Don had a difficult time finding his way around the house. I did my best to find ways to keep him involved in some way, to find ways for us to enjoy the time we had together. But as I worked at helping him get his pajamas on that Saturday night, his eyes met mine. Slowly and sadly his words came out.

"I feel like my mind is rotting . . . "

His words, the look on his face, broke my heart.

I knew that no verbal assurances could ease his pain, so with tears in my eyes and great sadness in my heart, I urged him to the safety of our own bed where we could simply curl up next to one another.

When we arrived at Wentworth Sunday evening, Don was not eager to enter the building. He reluctantly walked in the front door, down the hall, and through the glass corridor with me. But when we got to his room, shedding his coat became another hurdle to overcome. As confused as he had been at home, he had not objected to being there. Now he obviously knew this was not where he wanted to be.

Perhaps a walk, some exercise, a change of scenery, might help. Hand in hand, we walked and walked. We went up and down halls and corridors, took an elevator to the second floor, walked down the halls where the apartments were. As we rounded one corner, we suddenly found ourselves facing a cozy, private little nook with a comfortable-looking couch. Just what we needed.

We sat down. For a few moments, in that quiet corner of Wentworth, we simply sat together — in silence. Then, with downcast eyes, and a catch in his voice, those words came once again.

"I'm going to rot."

He paused, looked over at me, and then with that deep sadness still reflected in his eyes, in his face, in his voice, he said:

"I let you down . . ."

Those words were more than I could take.

My face crumpled with emotion and tears rolled down my cheeks — tears that had been building behind my smile — tears of fatigue, of tension, of great sorrow and sadness for us both. That night, I couldn't keep the words from rolling out.

"No. Never. You have never let me down!"

Over and over I told him that he was a special man, my special guy, that I loved him so very much — that we had always walked together, that we would now, that we would just take one day at a time.

We walked some more. I gave him a shower, washed his hair, got cookies and juice for both of us. Later I got him settled in bed, curled up next to him until he fell asleep, and then left for home.

Devastating thoughts and feelings raced through my mind and heart as I drove. I finally pulled into the garage, hurried into the house, and headed for the typewriter.

"I feel terrible — terrible about taking Don back to Wentworth tonight! I had wanted to bring him home. I thought it might be good for us both, that it might work again. But it was one time too many. I goofed! I should have known. He was so upset about returning. I should never have brought him back to the house this weekend. Somehow it made something click in his head, caused some memory to clear, reminded him that there was a different place — brought thoughts and feelings to his mind that he might have let me down! How awful! What an unbearable thing to have him think . . . or feel."

Even as these appalling thoughts were racing through my mind, another equally disturbing one suddenly burst into my consciousness. "Maybe I am letting him down by not being able to keep him at home, by utilizing a facility!"

I struggled to type my thoughts and emotions into the typewriter — feeling completely overwhelmed.

Slowly, my vision cleared.

I knew what Don Miller would say to those last thoughts. There was no question in my mind. We had lived together too long, shared too many thoughts and feelings, experienced too many things together over the years, for me not to know. He would say to me, "No. Never. You have never let me down."

It was all right. I was doing the very best I could, the very best I knew how, to travel this unbelievable road with him, to be there for him. And I knew he was not "happy" anywhere — even when he was home.

And although Don had not said anything about "home," for my own sake I needed to remember a comment that David had made one day — that when a loved one who has any form of dementia expresses the desire to "go home," "home" is not always the building or place we think they may be talking about. It is often a place, in his or her mind, where everything used to be "normal" and "safe."

Suddenly it all seemed like just too much. I stopped typing, and just sat. I felt absolutely exhausted. My thoughts continued to churn. Slowly, ever so slowly, a deep sense that I must relinquish the entire scene began to fill my being. I turned off the typewriter and mechanically walked upstairs to bed.

Early the next morning, with a lump in my throat, a heavy heart, and deep concern, I headed for Wentworth. What would I find when I arrived? My imagination could depict scenarios of all kinds, and it was difficult to contain my thoughts as I drove along.

Don was up. He was not only up, he was dressed, shaved, and his hair was neatly combed. He was seated in a comfortable chair in the adult home's small lounge, next to one of the women residents who had often spoken to me when I visited. She greeted me with a warm smile. She and Don were enjoying a snack, and watching the morning news. Don's grin of welcome warmed my heart and dissolved the lump in my throat. He looked content, and seemed delighted to see me.

"Is this your wife?" his amiable companion cheerfully asked Don. Almost to my surprise, he happily acknowledged that fact, although I wondered if he really understood her query. I quickly knelt down beside the two of them when I realized that Don was attempting to stand to greet me.

An aide pulled up a chair for me and offered to get me a cup of tea. Another woman resident with a walker arrived to join us, and the four of us were soon engaged in an exchange of friendly small talk. Don was not really able to participate, but seemed happy to be part of the cheerful group.

Those compassionate women who lived in the adult home continued to reach out to Don with love and concern over the next months. There were also people on the staff who began to understand and care about him. As I left for home one night, I stopped in the hall to talk with Donna, one of those special aides.

"I am getting to know Don," she said. "Even though he has a difficult time expressing himself, I can tell when he comes up to me, sort of wringing his hands, that he wants something. I can usually figure out what it is.

"And he seems to notice when I'm off for the day," she added. "I love his enthusiastic greeting when I come back!"

And there was the man who drove the facility's bus, and the delightful activity director. Both of these men always had a friendly greeting for Don, and went the "extra mile" to help him.

Throughout this new and larger facility, we were finding friends among the residents and staff.

I began to feel better about our move to Wentworth.

Residents from the apartments, the adult home, and those who were able from the nursing home, all ate in shifts in the large, formal dining room. At mealtime it was almost always filled with people. Often I stayed to eat with Don, but a spare seat was difficult to come by. There was a cafeteria for the staff and visitors, and I asked if it would be possible for us to occasionally eat our meals there.

The man in charge of the dining room crew responded with caring sincerity. "Anytime," he said with a warm smile. "I can arrange to have one of the tables in a corner by the window set up just for the two of you."

He did just that every time I asked, and it was always set just as nicely as those in the dining room — with a cloth tablecloth and napkins, and flowers carefully placed in the center of the table. He even provided our own private waiter each time we ate there. Those young men and women would cheerfully work both our little table, and those in the main dining room. How I appreciated that extra effort, those thoughtful gestures, and the young people whose smiling faces appeared at our table on the evenings that we took advantage of his offer.

On several occasions, some special friends of ours came over to join us at our "private" dinner table. I was very grateful for the company of good friends who would come to that facility, join us for a meal, and later graciously sit with us in Don's room in our little corner of Wentworth to "chat." I think Don enjoyed the diversion — and their compassion and understanding, their caring presence, meant a great deal to me.

About a month after Don moved to Wentworth, Sandy and her daughter Katie flew up for a brief visit. How wonderful it was to see their smiling faces, to watch that exuberant two-year-old bounce around the house, to share my thoughts and feelings with Sandy. We drove over to spend time with Don each day. His look of excitement, of joy, when the three of us walked up to him in the lounge was unbelievably heartwarming. Once again, I was not at all sure that he knew exactly who I was, or who they were, but how eagerly he embraced, and welcomed us.

We were talking in Don's room one afternoon, and had our *My Fair Lady* tape playing quietly in the background. That tape and movie had always been a favorite of Don's and mine, and one that Sandy, too, dearly loved. Obviously Katie had heard those delightful melodies and words played frequently in her home. She had been peering around and exploring the little room, when all of a sudden she climbed up on the bed where Don and I were sitting side by side. She placed a small arm on each of our shoulders. Then with a huge satisfied grin she looked over at her mom, who was sitting in Don's lounge chair, and said, "My fair ladies!" Sandy and I burst into warm, appreciative laughter, and Don soon joined the merriment. Katie grinned happily — then hopped down to continue her exploring.

What fun it was for all of us to be together — for Don to have time with Sandy and Katie, and for Sandy and Katie to have time with him.

Gradually the days became smoother for Don at Wentworth, but there were still times when I received calls saying he was agitated, that they didn't know how to deal with him. I would hurry over, and help ease his frustration or anger.

I was doing fairly well at keeping my own emotions under control amidst these daily challenges, but planning for some sad realities and difficult matters that would have to be faced in the future threatened to unnerve me.

I called the Alzheimer's Association and asked for forms to fill out to donate Don's brain for research when he died. The information on the sheets I received stressed that it was important to make arrangements in advance, as time was a crucial factor. So I called our local hospital to arrange for an autopsy after Don's death. Next, I called, then visited a local funeral home to make funeral and cremation arrangements.

These actions caused all kinds of new mental gyrations. Don was going to die. I was saying that they could cut out his brain and analyze it, with the hope that it would help others. I was saying they could burn his body. How was I really going to be able to deal with such things?

"You will be ready . . . " David said quietly.

I wasn't so sure . . .

Late in April, I realized that I was not getting as many calls about problems with Don. His care at Wentworth seemed to have stabilized, and I was grateful. I began to ease up in my efforts to spend part of each day with him. I always stopped by to say "hello" when I was in the area, but started going over to see him every other day on a regular basis. The point of utilizing a facility was to give me the time that I desperately needed. I began to consider the possibility of visiting both daughters, and in late May I made arrangements for a quick trip South. I carefully left numbers where I could be reached.

I had been gone four days, and was thoroughly enjoying the warmer weather, the change of pace, the time with our daughters and their families. Then the ring of the telephone changed everything. It was a long-distance call, for me, from the R.N. in charge of the adult unit at Wentworth. Don was very agitated. He was threatening to kill himself. He picked up a chair and they thought he was going to throw it. The other residents were afraid of him. He had told the R.N. that she was a "prostitute running a whore house."

Her call surprised and upset me, and as I listened to her reports, I became more and more concerned. Then suddenly my mind locked in on "a prostitute running a whore house . . ." An interesting choice of words on Don's part, I thought, as a picture of the whole scenario quickly flashed through my mind. I could almost envision his frustration, his growing anger . . . and his struggle to express his feelings. Then suddenly, in spite of myself, an inward chuckle started to build — and was probably reflected in my voice . . . The R.N.'s last statement began to sound absolutely ludicrous to me.

The complete silence at the other end of the phone let me know that she was deadly serious.

I said I would head back as soon as I was able to get a seat on a plane.

But even by flying "standby," the first airline seat available was not until the next evening. I sat on the plane staring out the window. The view was a magnificent one, as the setting sun in the west reflected its pink rays on the towering mountains of luminous white clouds.

The flight was smooth.

Only my thoughts bounced around.

What on earth would I find when I got to Wentworth?

I arrived too late. I quickly learned that the Wentworth staff had sent Don to the hospital — this time to the psychiatric unit!

Chapter Eight

Hospital visiting hours were over when I arrived at Wentworth, but I was able to talk my way into the psychiatric unit. I was tired from the long trip, and the strain and worry about what I would find. The sights and reports that awaited me slowly eroded what composure I had left.

I found Don in the hall, restrained in a "geri-chair," a wheel chair that has a large tray surrounding it, especially designed to keep a person confined. His eyes were glazed and staring, his hair disheveled. He barely registered my presence.

A staff member who noticed my arrival quickly approached me and quietly filled me in on what had happened.

Don had obviously become very upset about something. The staff on duty at Wentworth had attempted to control him physically. When that didn't work, they called for an ambulance to take him to the hospital's psych unit.

Don's frustration could have built over any number of things. I was well aware that he became frightened when people forcibly tried to control him. I knew that fear causes the adrenalin to flow in our bodies, and can cause the "fight or flight" syndrome to take over. Feeling confused, and physically unable to flee, I wondered if Don was "fighting" in the only way remaining to him — by getting angry — which was seen as "agitation" or "violence."

How logical it seemed that his fear could have turned to anger, and escalated when he found himself being put in a strange vehicle. I could certainly understand that he would have fought back.

The scenario presented to me was upsetting enough, but when I learned he had been "four-point" restrained en route, with both wrists and both ankles strapped down, I was angry! Angry at everybody and everything! Angry at myself for having left Don. Angry that some situation at Wentworth had been allowed to escalate and somehow end with his being sent to the psychiatric unit. Angry that no one was able to find other ways to help him, that anyone would have felt it necessary to restrain him in such a manner! Angry at Alzheimer's — angry at the world!

I asked the hospital staff personnel to please help me get Don out of that geri-chair, and down the hall to his room. We settled him into bed, and I did fairly well until the hospital nurse left. Then . . . as I sat there beside the bed in that psychiatric unit . . . the magnitude of the entire situation truly registered. Suddenly, all the feelings that had been building since I received the phone call seemed to completely overwhelm me. I laid my head on Don's chest and dissolved into tears.

Somehow . . . I drove myself home that night . . .

When I arrived the next morning, I learned that the hospital psychiatrist was conferring with David, and that they had decided to take Don off all medication in order to try something new. Together, they were searching for something different that might help with agitation and anger, as well as balance and coordination. Both doctors asked for my feedback, shared their thoughts, and took the time to explain what they were trying to do, and why — gestures which I greatly appreciated.

Their efforts eventually paid off, but for the next two days, Don's balance was so poor that he remained in the geri-chair most of the time. He was definitely not combative, but he was very confused, could not seem to get words out that made any sense at all, and much of the time just sat staring.

When I arrived the morning of the second day, the hospital charge nurse came up to me with a small manila envelope. It was labeled "Mr. Miller's Wedding Ring." Don had lost a fair amount of weight over recent months, and the ring had become loose on his finger. She saw him taking it off and on . . . off and on, was afraid it might get lost, and had quietly tucked it away in the little envelope to save and give to me.

With a catch in my voice I said, "Thank you . . . " How easily that priceless little circle of gold could have been lost forever.

I slipped the familiar smooth gold ring onto my finger. It nestled up against my own ring, and soon felt warm . . . and strangely comforting.

A meeting was arranged at the hospital with the charge nurse on the psych unit, the hospital's social worker, their female psychiatrist, and the R.N. in charge of Wentworth's adult home. I asked Mike to come with me, to help listen to what was being said.

After we had discussed the whole situation and Don's current status, the R.N. from Wentworth said they could no longer keep Don in the adult home. They did not have enough supervision, and their staff was not trained to work with someone who became combative. She said they did have a bed in the nursing home.

I went to see Don during every scheduled visiting time, traveling back and forth between our home and the hospital twice a day. Gradually, he began to look better, and seemed a little more "clear." I would wash his hair, brush his teeth, shave him, and change his clothes. Hand in hand, we began to walk slowly up and down the hospital halls.

Late Friday afternoon, June 11, the R.N. from Wentworth's adult home called to say that now they had no available beds in the nursing home section. She reiterated that they would not take him back into their adult home — he was violent, combative, and they could not handle him. They would put Don's things in a storage room until I picked them up.

All of a sudden no bed?

How could it be that things had gone so smoothly while Don was at Sunnybrook, but less than two months after his move to Wentworth he was considered violent, combative, unmanageable, and a candidate for the psych unit?

Don was not someone with a severe psychiatric problem. He had Alzheimer's disease! I knew that the progression of the disease can cause rapid, radical, and unexpected changes in a person's behavior. I also knew that the manner in which a person responds to that behavior has a great deal to do with the responses received.

There were people on the staff in Wentworth's adult home area who had grown to care about Don, and who were able to help him through the rough times with great skill. But I had noticed that there were others who did not do as well, and who did not seem to want to try.

I was well aware that I had much to learn, and was discovering that some people who are professional caregivers could also benefit from learning more about helping people who suffer with Alzheimer's disease.

Early the next week, I spoke with Wentworth's social worker — the person in charge of admissions. I suggested that if they admitted Don to the nursing home unit, we could all work together. I told her I was readily available to help, and suggested that perhaps all of us might continue to learn from this situation.

She didn't agree.

"He doesn't belong in our facility," she told me bluntly.

Then where, I wondered, did Don Miller "belong?"

How I wished that things were different — that he was back to normal — that he truly belonged at home with me. But I knew that was not the reality — that it could never again be the reality for Don, or for me.

Back and forth we went with words. Back and forth I went from the hospital to the nursing home. And back and forth I drove between the hospital, Wentworth, and our home.

I had looked at many facilities, chosen the best one that I could find in our area, and I did not want to move Don again.

I talked further with the hospital social worker, with the hospital psychiatrist, and with David about what to do. I met with Wentworth's administrator — told him how impressed we had been with their facility, how we had chosen Wentworth over many others, and why. I reiterated that I would continue to be active in helping with Don's care. Surely together we could find ways to help Don. And I reminded him that part of the reason I chose Wentworth over other facilities was the fact that a person admitted to their adult home had "priority access" to their nursing home.

"But Don is a very difficult person with whom to deal," he said, repeating what both their R.N. and social worker had said. He paused, then finally continued.

"Why don't you go back and talk with the hospital psychiatrist, see what her thoughts are, and call me."

So, back I went to Brentwood Hospital.

"I do feel that Don is ready to be discharged," the psychiatrist said thoughtfully, "but I agree with the idea that he is no longer appropriate for Wentworth's adult home. I will talk with the people at Wentworth."

That afternoon while I was still at the hospital, I called the administrator at Wentworth. He put the social worker on the phone.

"We can admit Don to our nursing home section on Thursday," she said. Now, a bed had suddenly become available.

When I told the hospital psychiatrist about the latest development, she looked me straight in the eye and quietly said: "It would not have happened without your advocating for Don."

I went to the hospital social worker's office to share the news. She stood up and shook my hand.

I was never completely sure, and did not ponder much about what caused the people at Wentworth to reverse their decision. I was grateful for the fact that there was now space available, and grateful that they had decided to readmit Don. What was important was Don's care — and in my mind at that point in time, there was no question that Wentworth was the very best place he could be.

Mike went over to Wentworth, retrieved Don's things from the storage room, and set up the new room.

When we arrived at Wentworth, the compassionate activity director was at the door with a warm smile of greeting. Over and over, I had watched that man's efforts to include Don in activities, watched him find ways to help Don cope, watched his consistent efforts to simply let Don know that he cared.

A little later, Wentworth's driver appeared at the door of Don's new room with a big grin and cheerful welcome. How many times I had noticed that kind and gentle man go out of his way to greet, talk with, and befriend Don, even though Don was unable to participate in outside trips or activities and had never ridden in Wentworth's private shuttle bus.

I much appreciated the thoughtfulness of these two men, and was so very grateful for the fact that they, and other friends in the facility, would be there caring for and about Don, even though he would now be in the nursing home section.

I was unbelievably tired, but ever so thankful to have Don back at Wentworth. I knew the facility had a fine reputation. I was still frustrated about what had happened in the adult home — but perhaps now he did require more skilled care than that group had been trained to give. I felt certain the people on the staff in the nursing home would be better equipped to help him.

And they were. Teresa, a kind, friendly, perceptive Licensed Practical Nurse (L.P.N.) immediately reached out to both Don and me.

"From the way Don responds to you, and the way you treat him, I can tell that you two have a very loving relationship," she said to me one day. "I really love Don too," she continued, "And I am learning so much about how to help him just by watching you."

How awesome to hear. Her candid words put a glow in my heart. It was gratifying to know that as I learned ways to help Don, I might also be able to help someone else learn.

Martha, a pretty, dark-haired, young R.N., also did especially well with Don, and became a loyal supporter. And there were other members of this new staff who began to care about Don, who seemed to understand how to help him.

Quick movements and loud demanding voices could surprise or frighten him, and cause an abrupt reaction. Soft tones and slow and careful movements, could work wonders. Talking about him as one worked, or talking "around" him as if he were not there, obviously bothered Don, and bothered me as well.

Alzheimer's disease was limiting his abilities in many areas, but it was obvious that he still had feelings. In spite of bouts with agitation and anger, Don would often reflect and respond positively to compassion. Patience, understanding, and respect could penetrate the wall of Alzheimer's and become powerful tools in helping him.

I arrived at Wentworth late one morning in June and found Don up, dressed, and quietly sitting in a chair in the lounge. We took a walk, and later had lunch in his room. When one of the aides came in to get our trays and talk to Don for a few moments, I suddenly noticed Martha standing just outside the door. She smiled, and silently beckoned to me.

I met her in the hall, and we moved a few steps away from the door to talk.

"There's something I want to tell you," she said quietly. "Yesterday morning I noticed that Don was frustrated, and becoming quite agitated. The aides that were on didn't know him very well and couldn't seem to help him, so when I had a bit of free time, I urged him to go for a walk with me. As we moved up and down the hall together, he said, 'Why is this happening to me? I'm an intelligent man . . .'

"I felt so badly," she told me softly.

We looked at one another in silence, as the deep sadness of that moment flooded over us both . . .

There were times when Don was fairly cheerful, when we could joke with him, and even get him to laugh. And how rewarding it was when we succeeded in getting him over a hurdle, when we could help him find that cheerful manner, that grin that always warmed my heart. But overall, things continued to move downhill that summer of 1993. His frustration often resulted in continuous pacing up and down the halls. His balance was poor, causing all of us to be concerned about the possibility of his falling. When he withdrew unto himself, he appeared to be off in another world. Often that other world was one of the past . . .

Early one afternoon I got a call from Teresa.

"Oh, Pat," she said with relief in her voice, "I'm so glad you are home. Don has been in tears all morning. He is remembering that he is a runner, an engineer, and seems to know that he belongs somewhere else.

"He seems to feel so lost and alone," she continued, "and keeps saying no one loves him. We have all been in tears, too. We keep telling him that Pat loves him . . . that we love him . . . and trying and trying to help. Finally, I told him I would call Pat. Could you come?"

Could I come? Of course. And I hurried over.

The use of a toilet became less and less comprehensible to Don, and he began wearing adult diapers. It broke my heart to realize that he seemed very aware that he was having trouble. It was deeply upsetting to him, and he would object strongly to having others change those diapers regularly. There were times when he understandably became upset and angry. How hurtful it was for him to be aware — but not to understand. Yet . . . true understanding of the situation we were in might have been equally devastating.

And on my part . . . although I had read many things about the various stages of this disease, about things that might happen, about what to expect . . . I wondered, can a caregiver ever really be prepared for the challenges that may lie ahead? I'm not at all sure we can. But I do know that for anyone walking down a similar, or even a very different path, however unprepared or ill-equipped we may feel for what comes our way, we deal the very best we can.

I continued to visit regularly, usually staying part of the afternoon and into the evening. Sometimes I would lie down beside Don when he went to bed, and wait for him to fall asleep. Then I would inch my body away from his, and try to slip off that hospital bed without disturbing him. There would be times when his hand would suddenly grip my arm, and hang on to it with his firm grasp. I would wait until that hand relaxed, until those eyes stayed closed, until that familiar face relaxed. Only then would I head for home.

The weeks rolled into months, and before long summer was almost over. I was hesitant to visit our daughters, hesitant to travel anywhere except between our home and where Don was. I spent many hours on the telephone with Sandy and Lisa, as I kept them posted, and their caring voices and loving thoughts supported me. Our phone bills were enormous, and worth every penny.

One evening in late August, I was sitting in my comfortable lounge chair in the living room, engrossed in a book.

The doorbell rang. I glanced at my watch. It was 9:30 p.m. One of our neighbors? I eased up out of the chair, walked to the front door, and peered through the tiny peephole. I could see nothing but the porch, and the bushes on either side. I carefully turned the knob, pulled the door open a few inches, and leaned around to see who was there.

No one. Was I "hearing things?"

Then my glance dropped down a few feet. A little person. A little girl. Slim, blonde, pretty. Katie?! Yes! There stood Katie, with a huge grin spreading across her small face.

Katie. She and her mom and dad live in North Carolina. If there is a Katie on my front porch, there must be a Sandy, my sluggish mind began to reason.

"Surprise!" rang out of the darkness, followed by three cheerful voices singing, "Happy Birthday to you, Happy Birthday to you . . . "

From behind the bushes on either side of the porch suddenly emerged not one, but two figures — Sandy and Lisa!

I just stood there . . . my head still not registering the joyous event.

Sandy. Katie. And Lisa? Lisa and her husband live in Virginia . . . How could they all be here at my front door?

Birthday? My birthday is not until Saturday! It took me a while, as we stood there on the front porch, laughing and hugging.

Amidst the jumble of words, the story began to come out. My birthday was coming. What could they do for me? Telephone calls sometimes seemed so mundane on a special occasion. Flowers? Candy? Aha! This year they would come! They would both come. Together. And they would surprise me.

They definitely succeeded!

As I stood there with a silly grin on my face, savoring the joy of the moment, Sandy and Lisa reveled in my surprise and amazement, in the success of their venture. How very often over the days ahead I was to remember that marvelous present our two thoughtful, loving daughters had given me during those difficult times.

The hours we spent with Don over the next two days were filled with mixed emotions. We were so glad to be together, and grateful that Don enjoyed the visits, whether or not he was able to recognize exactly who we all were. But it was always difficult for the girls to see the dramatic changes in Don each time they visited. It was painfully apparent to each of us that he was moving inexorably downhill.

When I arrived at Wentworth one evening after Sandy, Lisa, and Katie had returned to their homes, I discovered Mike was visiting Don. I spotted the two of them walking down the hall toward me when I first entered the nursing home area. I stopped in my tracks. Usually I was the one who walked with Don down that hall, and what a shock it was to see them from the observer perspective.

I just stood there watching. I was having trouble registering what I saw. Don was almost leaning on Mike's big frame, as they slowly moved toward me. He looked so old — and to me he seemed so young. The reality shook me, and I hurried toward them with a grin, trying to shake the vision.

But there were some special times — some heartwarming occasions that could sometimes help soften the effects of the devastatingly negative aspects of our walk.

Like the scene one evening as I walked up and down the halls with Don. An older woman who was confined to a wheelchair reached out to us saying, "Please, Honey . . . " as she often did. That night, Don stopped. He slowly reached his hand toward her, gently touched her arm, looked into her face with obvious concern, and smiled. He was so mixed up himself, yet how graciously he tried to respond to her need in his sincere, friendly, manner. I squeezed his hand with love and respect, and walked a bit taller myself, as we moved on down the hallway.

One bright September afternoon, I took him outside. We sat side by side on a bench, soaking up the autumn sun. Gradually, the shadows began to lengthen, and the sun's rays weakened. I began to feel chilled, and realized Don, too, might be getting cold. I urged him to stand, and we headed inside and down the hallway to his room.

I helped him get settled in his lounge chair, then jokingly sat down on his lap. He chuckled, ran his hands over my hair, cupped my face with his hands and sort of patted it, as he continued to grin at me. We sat like this for a while. When he appeared to be falling asleep, I urged him to lie down on his bed for a nap before dinner. On impulse, I lay down beside him. He carefully moved over a bit to give me more room, and painstakingly hooked his arm around mine.

On another pleasant afternoon, I was on my way out the door, then turned around and retraced my steps to where I had left Don sitting in the lounge with several other residents. For some reason on that particular day, I was more hesitant to leave than usual . . .

He was still sitting there in a comfortable chair, looking a bit glum. Suddenly he glanced up, looked my way as I approached, and with great enthusiasm and a huge grin of welcome burst out with, "There she is!"

How glad I was that I had walked back to where he was. I would not have missed that special greeting for anything.

Another evening, I left a little early to run some errands. When I came out of the mall, I decided I wanted to stop by to see Don on the way home, even though it was almost 10:00 p.m. Again, I found him sitting in the lounge, this time, all by himself. And again, I was so grateful I had followed my instincts and come back.

As I hurried toward him, he spotted me, and with obvious delight, he said, "Pat!"

That rare voicing of my name, that one-word exclamation, made with such unmistakable pleasure and excitement, brought a grin to my face, and tears to my eyes.

And there was the day I arrived to find Martha walking with Don in the hall. She spotted me, grinned with a cheerful and welcoming smile, and said to him:

"Who is this?"

"My heroine!" Don responded promptly.

His heroine . . .

I will never forget those tiny moments in time.

Chapter Nine

On September 20, 1993, the telephone rang in the middle of the night. I struggled to read the clock by the bed, groggily realized it was 4:30 a.m., and almost knocked the phone off the dresser in my attempts to get the receiver to my ear.

"This is the charge nurse at Wentworth," said the voice on the other end of the line. "Don is choking on water, we can't arouse him, and are taking him to the emergency room."

I was instantly alert, and could feel my heart suddenly pounding and my pulse racing. "I'll meet him there," I said in a hoarse voice. My feet hit the floor, and I hurriedly, and almost automatically, got dressed and headed for the hospital.

This time, it was pneumonia, and they admitted him.

That next evening I sat in a chair next to Don's hospital bed, holding his limp hand. He lay so still . . . The entire room was still. The IV tube dripped silently into his veins. Water. Glucose. Salt. Electrolytes. And antibiotics . . . to combat the pneumonia.

All of a sudden my thoughts clicked into action.

"Antibiotics? What are you doing using antibiotics to fight off pneumonia? Don is lying here absolutely helpless. You know how much he loves you, how much he trusts you. Is this what he would want you to do? How many, many times has he made it perfectly plain, perfectly clear to you, that he would rather die than live like a vegetable? And long before there were any signs of this disease, the two of you discussed death and dying, filled out health care proxy forms, and carefully worded your living wills.

"Someone else might think differently, but you know what Don Miller would want.

"Would you want antibiotics if the situation were reversed? Would he give them to you? He might struggle with the decision because of his love for you, but you know he would respect your wishes."

I quietly slipped my hand out of Don's, and headed down the hall toward the nursing station.

I would call Sandy, Lisa, and David. I needed their perspective, their inputs. A decision was beginning to form in my mind, but I needed support, and validation.

I asked if I could use the telephone.

It was late. Would I be able to reach David? Sandy and Lisa would be up. I would try David first. I pulled out my telephone card and started dialing.

I was relieved to find him at home.

"Follow your heart," he said. "Listen for guidance." He agreed. Perhaps this was an opportunity for Don to go free.

"Yes," said both Sandy and Lisa.

An enormous decision, but the answer seemed crystal clear. We should let nature take its course. We should keep Don comfortable and wait and see what happened. We should not try to fight pneumonia with antibiotics. If Don had been able to be part of the decision, we were certain that he would wholeheartedly concur.

My next call was to the attending physician at the hospital. Would he, could he, stop the antibiotics now that they had been started? Don's living will, and the fact that I was his health-care proxy, might help him support our decision. I found him, too, at home. After a bit of hesitation, he agreed. He would contact the hospital.

I had barely returned to Don's room when the R.N. on duty appeared to make the proper adjustments. On impulse, I asked for her thoughts, probably still seeking reinforcement for such a momentous decision. She paused for a moment, then smiled into my eyes and thoughtfully said, "I can't tell you what to do . . . "

"You're right . . . " I said slowly.

But later that night, the same young woman came in to see me. She quietly told me that she understood Don's situation, was well aware of the Alzheimer's diagnosis, and although she could never have advised me about what to do, she unreservedly supported our decision.

I thanked her from the bottom of my heart.

Then warmed by her words, I settled into the lounge chair by Don's bed . . . and waited.

We were alone.

The staff moved in and out of the room.

Stopping the antibiotics was one thing . . . but when Don's temperature crept up slowly, and finally reached 104 degrees, that was not something with which I could deal. I agreed to the suggestion of using Tylenol suppositories to try to bring it down.

The nurses laid a cooling pad under Don. They administered the Tylenol, suctioned his throat, and swabbed it to help with the irritation. They were kind and gentle as they worked to lower his temperature and keep him comfortable.

Slowly, his temperature began to drop. He had been admitted early Monday morning, and by Thursday it was down to 100 degrees, and staying there. He began to eat small amounts of food. Soon, he started greeting the nurses with a smile, and even laughed when they tried to joke with him.

I think it was a surprise to all of us that Don rallied.

I was glad.

I really was not ready to say "goodbye" . . .

On Friday afternoon, we were able to help him up, and the two of us slowly tried walking a little ways down the hall. As we haltingly moved up and down the hallways together over the next few days, the nurses all greeted us warmly. When we stopped the antibiotics, I think many of them thought that he would not make it. I hadn't been so sure myself. But as I felt the warmth of Don's hand in mine, watched him flash the familiar grin that melts my heart, I was grateful for his presence. I knew the decision had been the right one, and one we might make again. But nevertheless, I was grateful for the opportunity to be walking down halls once again.

By the following Tuesday, Don was eating fairly well, seemed to be stabilized, and received the okay to leave the hospital.

But about a week after we returned to Wentworth, he began to show no interest in food. He refused to take the new medication and antidepressant that David and the psychiatrist at Brentwood Hospital had agreed to try. Sometimes he just held things in his mouth, or nicely pushed the food away, or just looked at us and would not open his mouth. We couldn't tell if he was having a difficult time swallowing, if he couldn't figure out what to do with the food once it was in his mouth, or if he was semi-aware that he did not want to eat. For whatever reason, he was eating practically nothing.

One evening he was pleasant and cheerful, but would not eat his dinner. Later that night, I felt as though I should try again. I asked for a sandwich and a small chocolate sundae for him. He ate only a few bites of each.

In spite of very little food and hardly any medication, he remained in an unusually consistent good mood, almost "punch drunk" at times. Neither the agitation nor the anger arose as often.

The pattern continued, and one evening I gathered my courage. Don was lying on the bed — I was sitting in a little chair beside him. I slipped off the chair and knelt down beside the bed, so that I could touch him — be closer to him.

"You know, Honey, if you don't eat, you will continue to lose weight. Your body needs food and water. If you are conscious of wanting out of this situation, and if you are not eating for that reason, I understand. We have talked many times over the years about the idea that each of us may be something more than these physical bodies, that there may be something more beyond what we call 'death.' If you ever sense something more, a Light, a Love . . . anything that seems to beckon you on . . . it would be all right to go . . .. " As I spoke, tears filled my eyes. I told him I didn't want to lose him, but it was okay to go if that was his decision.

Could he possibly comprehend? He seemed to be listening intently. Was it right to say such things? I didn't know. The words just seemed to roll out that night.

Don was looking right at me, but when I stopped talking, he began to sort of search with his eyes, then appeared to be looking at something "beyond me." He almost seemed to be listening . . . to something. He looked at me again, with sort of a sidewise grin — then looked away. Suddenly he looked back, and with a great big grin, looked me straight in the eyes.

Then his grin became a gentle smile . . . and he slowly drifted off to sleep.

I suddenly realized how stiff I was getting as I knelt there on the floor. I eased myself back up to a standing position, leaned over, and gently kissed Don on the cheek. I stood, just looking . . . for a long time.

What if he was really hearing and understanding what I was saying? What if he was sensing something that I could not comprehend . . . and what if . . . he slipped away after I left . . .

I sat back down on the chair and watched. He seemed to be so relaxed . . . with that tender smile still lingering on his face. His breathing seemed easy. Should I leave? "Yes. Go," said my head. I finally tiptoed out, walked down the hall, out to the car, and headed home with tears in my eyes, wondering if Don would be there for me to visit in the morning.

He was. But over the next month, he continued to eat very little. He had lost 16 pounds since early September.

One evening as I tried to help him with dinner, he refused everything I offered. He just sat there, looking at me. I tried some mashed potatoes. He would not take them. Suddenly, he said, "Damn . . . Scary."

Did he truly know what he was doing when he said "no" to food? I simply could not know.

A little later that evening we sat together in his chair, listening to some of our favorite tapes. He seemed almost happy, and certainly content. Suddenly he said, "You're a trooper . . . you're tops." He paused, then looked at me closely and said, "What's your name?"

To my response of "Pat," he said, "Is that right!?" with a rather surprised, yet pleased look on his face.

What brief, but meaningful comments. What a purposeful question . . . and purposeful response. What was he thinking, and feeling?

Could he really comprehend why the name "Pat" brought him pleasure? I wasn't at all sure. Yet the awareness that I was someone very special to him continued to surface. He almost always reacted positively, and with great enthusiasm, when he first saw me each time I arrived, and there was no question that he responded differently to me than to the aides when I changed his diapers, gave him a shower, or helped in any such effort. I wondered if perhaps he sensed my approach, my touch, my love . . . or perhaps there is something that we just don't understand that joins us to loved ones . . .

Several times over the months and years, aides who seemed to be able to work very well with him, made the comment that he was more "there" than many people observed — that there was much more awareness than most people understood or believed. Those who really took the time and effort to try to "reach" Don were often surprised by what they found.

I still wonder if Don was capable of understanding the idea of not eating during that period of time. If he was truly aware, evidently that awareness was not something that could remain in his consciousness very long.

During the last weeks of October, he gradually became more interested in food. He began to eat a little for all of us, and began to pick items up on his own as well. He even appeared to relish what he was eating. One night when I was helping him, he ate small amounts and with great enthusiasm finished off the meal with a sundae!

He also began to accept the medications David and the doctor at Brentwood Hospital had prescribed.

One evening after dinner, we sat in Don's room together. He was sitting in his lounge chair, and I had pulled our little chair up beside him. Once again he was looking at me closely, and seemed unusually aware of my presence. It caught me off guard, and I could feel the tears welling up in my eyes. It seemed like a long time since his eyes had seemed so perceptive, since they had been turned in my direction with such intensity.

As, one by one, the tears started slowly rolling down my cheeks, Don appeared very concerned.

My thoughts and feelings came rolling out. "I love you so much, Honey . . . I know you love me. You are a wonderful husband, friend, dad . . ."

He reached his hand out and gently wiped the tears from my cheeks. He patted my arm . . . and reached over to hug me. Then slowly, and with deep feeling, the man who could often be perceived only as demented, as violent, by those who had trouble seeing beyond their visual perceptions, said:

"Thank you."

My guy was in there somewhere.

And he loved me.

Don began to have more trouble keeping his balance that winter of 1993-94. Walking hand in hand was adequate at times, but I found a way to place my left arm across his waist to grasp his left hand, my right arm across my waist to grasp his right hand. That "skating position" provided the added support he needed.

Along with his deteriorating mobility problems, there were more occasions when Don became frustrated and angry. Seeking to find a way to help everyone over those bumps, David had ordered one of the prescribed medications PRN (Pro Re Nata), meaning it was to be used whenever necessary, and at the staff's discretion, to de-fuse the situation if Don's feelings erupted.

I continued to visit regularly, stay for extended periods, and to hurry over when the staff called. I was fairly comfortable with the care Don was getting at Wentworth, and was not prepared for what happened late one January afternoon in 1994.

I was asked to meet with Wentworth's social worker. A brief discussion about Don's problems led quickly to "incident" reports that she said had been filed with the charge nurse when various staff members had difficulty working with Don. She added that as his capabilities deteriorated, his frustration level was rising, and many staff members were "afraid of him." She concluded with the rather ominous-sounding statement, that they would send Don to the psych unit again, if they found they could not "handle" him.

I was completely surprised and taken aback by the adamant tone of her voice, surprised by the attitude that reflected Don as such a "serious problem" — surprised that they were documenting every difficulty they encountered in what they called "incident" reports. I struggled to repress the anger that had begun to build as soon as she suggested sending Don back to the hospital psych unit. The possibility of his being four-point restrained once again, was something I would not tolerate!

"Please don't send him back to the psychiatric unit," I urged, as calmly as I could. "I have purchased a cell phone so that your staff can reach me at all times. Please call me if difficulties arise. I will come immediately."

She agreed.

So they called.

Four days later the call was from Bernice, the L.P.N. in charge of the floor that morning. Don hit her, she reported, and broke her stethoscope! Later he threw orange juice, squashed a muffin and threw it at her! She had him restrained in a geri-chair, and he was angry, rattling it violently.

"I'm going to call the psych unit," she declared.

"Please wait . . ." I pleaded, and immediately hurried over to calm Don.

A few days later, the phone rang early in the morning. It was the R.N. who was in charge of the floor on that day. Don was very angry. He had "threatened" one of the ladies.

I left the stack of paperwork I had just started to work on . . . and headed for Wentworth.

The descriptions often became quite graphic. On one occasion, the report was that Don was running down the hall after an aide . . . and that he had no clothes on!

With each incident, I would hurry over. I began to spend even more time at Wentworth than I had previously. I listened. I watched. Problems seemed to arise at predictable times. Obviously things were better when I was around, but also, it seemed as though Don's frustration level often had a great deal to do with which staff members were on duty.

Some people took the time to get to know Don, truly cared about him, and worked well with him. Some did not. There was no question in my mind that he responded more positively to those who took those extra minutes, found the extra patience, and reflected warmth and respect.

I had been so involved with trying to work with Don's changing abilities, trying to work along with the staff, trying to keep up with all the things that demanded attention in our personal lives, trying to deal with my own emotions . . . that I had been missing the developing undertones. Two things slowly began to dawn on me.

The first was that the administrative people were not as ready as I was to search for solutions to Don's problems, and were definitely ready to send him back to the psychiatric unit.

Secondly, I began to sense that in regard to Don's care, there was a growing division between various staff members who worked on the unit itself. There were occasions when animosity between them would surface and quietly filter back to me.

Suddenly things came to a head. One morning in mid-January, I received a telephone call from the doctor who worked with patients at Wentworth. He said that the administrative personnel considered Don a "problem resident," and were not sure they wanted him at Wentworth any longer.

After we hung up, it took a few moments for his comment to truly register. The administrative people at Wentworth were not only ready to send Don to the psychiatric unit when problems arose, but also they weren't even sure they wanted him in their facility! In retrospect, I suppose the comment should not have surprised me. But on that morning, my brain was simply not computing the situation from their perspective.

After the call, I hurried over to Wentworth. When I walked into the lounge, I found Don still in his nightshirt, with chinos pulled over the top of it. He was unshaven, very wet, and obviously upset.

"He wouldn't let us change him. He almost hit me, and he kicked a male aide!" I was informed when I arrived.

I looked around. None of our favorite people were on duty that day.

I took Don's hand, and walked back to his room with him. Although he was a little agitated with me at first, it was not that difficult to calm him, clean him up, get him into dry clothes, and shave him. I got him settled in his chair, and smiled at him. As I looked at the "new" Don, I was grateful for the staff members who could work with him, and deeply frustrated with those who could not.

The situation escalated further. The ominous warnings delivered by Wentworth's social worker and doctor were followed a few days later by a new development. I was asked to attend a meeting at Wentworth scheduled for January 19, 1994.

When I told David about the upcoming meeting, he suggested that I ask for their permission to tape it. He would not be able to attend, and that record might help him understand what was going on — what their main difficulties were — and how better to prescribe medication and provide suggestions about how to respond to certain behaviors.

With the knowledge and permission of the group, I taped the meeting. I have listened and relistened to that tape, and typed the words verbatim into my computer. The Wentworth social worker was there. The charge nurse from Don's unit was there. The activity director, the dietitian, the occupational therapist, and several others who were involved with Don's care were present. The activity director and the occupational therapist appeared to be the only truly supportive members of the group. I was grateful for their presence.

The following are matters discussed at the meeting, and any words in quotation marks are taken directly from that tape.

"Would you like for me to take some notes for you?" the occupational therapist asked thoughtfully. I gratefully accepted her offer.

The charge nurse began by going over many aspects of Don's condition, and carefully laid out the group's perspective of the situation. Don's cognitive and communicative skills were deteriorating. His gait was unsteady. A staff member would accompany him as often as possible. He tended to wander, and they were using the anklet connected to the alarm system to warn staff if he went out the main door.

Bathing and dressing were major difficulties, especially in the morning. It seemed as though anxiety and agitation were exacerbated by his incontinence. They used a geri-chair to restrain him at times, and found that he tolerated it better than they had expected. They were trying to work with the staff to help them maintain safety for him and themselves.

"Don picks up very quickly on behavioral cues that we might give him," the occupational therapist quietly inserted, "like if we are afraid, or if there is any hesitancy on our part."

"No question," I quickly agreed.

There was a pause in the discussion, then the charge nurse continued. "We need an emergency plan. In case of an emergency, we will send Don to Brentwood Hospital's Mental Health Unit, if we are unable to calm him down."

Brentwood . . . the psych unit . . . I could feel my inner anger building.

"I have requested a number of times, and I think people are pretty aware of it, that rather than calling Brentwood immediately, please call me," I said quietly. "I have purchased a cell phone which I always have with me. I can almost always calm him."

"You are right at the top of the list," responded the social worker. "But we have to have a crisis plan in place in case Don becomes aggressive and cannot be managed, and there is a real safety issue for our residents and staff. You have been wonderful about coming, but you are 20 minutes away — in good weather . . . There has to be something for the staff to do, especially in the evenings or on weekends, when we have less staff. Then we would have to call the mental health unit."

"What is difficult," I said, "is that several times they have called, said things were really bad, I have asked them to wait, and by the time I get here he has calmed down. Often things seem to be a 'crisis,' we all panic, then he calms down. I do appreciate it when they have called me," I continued, trying to measure my words and not allow my growing feelings of anger to take over.

"The staff would like to continue to do that," responded the social worker, "but we have to look at what is happening, who is getting hurt, and how often — because the staff is really getting hurt! No one feels that the mental health unit is the best place for someone with Don's diagnosis; it's just a matter of where the best place really is where the staff has the training so that they can handle the behavior and other parts of the dementia. That's what I have been working on — trying to call different places, different specialists, and ask what's being done. I have a list of places we can go over where they have Alzheimer's-specific programs dealing with severe behavior, unpredictable behavior, which is the category Don is falling into at this point."

"But if we could learn to help Don, all of us — I am learning, and it seems as though others are learning too. You must have had others, and will have more people who have Alzheimer's disease and who are agitated," I suggested. "Don is an intelligent man, a gentle man. He's not an aggressive person. It's the disease! And if we could learn how to help him, we would all gain."

"What we are hearing from the behavior specialists with whom we are consulting," continued the social worker, "is that the way we train staff for our nursing home is not sufficient training for someone with severe behavior. The staff on a psychiatric unit goes through specialized training that gives them the ability to manage someone with unpredictable episodes of aggression. I'm not talking about manacles and four-point restraint, I'm talking about different ways to protect themselves as well as the person who is being aggressive. Since our staff is not trained that way, we are having problems."

"I used to work at the Medical Hospital on the psych unit," interjected another woman, "and there were several patients who had that same type of episodic and aggressive behavior. They would use a padded room."

"We don't . . . we don't have that," the social worker responded.

"Behavior specialists . . . Padded room . . . Perhaps what we really need is more consistent simple acts of kindness, more patience, more compassion," I thought to myself.

"What I find with Don," I said quietly, "is that if he is walking down the hall and angry, sometimes I have just walked up, slipped my hand in his, and walked with him. Or when he is angry and lashing out, I just say, 'It's okay, we'll stop; let's just sit for a minute.' If we stop and I divert him, or we sit down somewhere, his agitation almost always seems to ease up. I know he's my husband, that I have a different relationship with him, but I think it's kind of how one goes at some of this. It's not to criticize anybody, but we're all learning. I'm learning too."

"I think that the issue we are facing now is that we can't really give him care without somebody getting hurt," the charge nurse reiterated. "Some other residents have sporadic agitation, but with Don, it is so predictable. It's been hard for us to really do him justice, to give him care. We are faced with giving him care and someone getting hurt, or just leaving him alone, which means neglecting him. And we don't really want to have to do that. Was there anything else?" she asked, looking at the social worker.

"I think we're all in agreement," the social worker responded. "I guess what I feel is that we need to at least start exploring alternative placement where they have behavior specialists, Alzheimer's specialists, and have them start doing assessments, paperwork."

Alternative placement? Assessments and paperwork? They were not simply unsure about wanting to keep Don at Wentworth. Now they were deciding to investigate other facilities for him . . . without even consulting me.

I could hardly believe what I was hearing. Yet it seemed that challenging the statement would do nothing but create more discord. Finally, I repeated my earlier thoughts.

"It still seems to me that the more we can all learn about this, the more that everybody wins."

"But right now, I don't feel Don is winning," the social worker responded. "When the staff is running from him in fear, which some staff are doing . . ."

"But to run in fear is going to make things worse," I suggested.

"And that's what we're telling them. But I worry about how this must be affecting Don, to see fear all around him. I would feel . . . it would bother me if I were in his position," she responded.

"But Don is the most gentle man I've ever known. It's the disease . . ." I said.

"I think everyone agrees that he is a wonderful person, but . . ." replied the charge nurse.

" . . . and if Wentworth," I continued, "with the outstanding reputation that your facility has, says 'Okay, we can't deal with Alzheimer's disease,' who's going to? And what are you going to do when you have more Alzheimer's patients who come and apply?"

"I think we still need to learn," the social worker acknowledged, "to keep on learning, because there's no quick solution to what we are dealing with now. But to answer your question, I think we need to look more at how we are admitting people to begin with. I mean if somebody is — if we know that they are likely to have aggressive behavior — we might have to say that we can't take them."

"But it's the disease!" I repeated helplessly, almost adding, "that causes certain behavior, and the manner in which some of your caregivers respond to that behavior can make the situation even more difficult."

But I didn't add that last comment. I paused, then asked in a voice that obviously reflected my sense of helplessness.

"So are you basically saying you want me to move Don out?"

"I think we need to explore that," responded the social worker.

Finally . . . I was out of words. I just sat there, feeling unbelievably frustrated and defeated, trying to assimilate the ideas that were being expressed, trying to understand . . .

"I hope you know," I said slowly, "that this is an emotional thing for me. Don is the most important person in my life. He is a kind, gentle, intelligent, athletic, 64-year-old man. It could happen to any of us . . . any of you. And I came here because you have a marvelous reputation. It was the only place I could find that I thought 'I can have my guy come here . . . ' So, I guess I'm disappointed. But . . . ah, we'll deal one way or another, with or without you."

A long pause follows on my tape . . .

"I just can't imagine the kind of agony you are going through. Such a difficult situation," the occupational therapist said quietly. "I don't think any of us are feeling very good about how this is going — for us, or for you. It's just such a hard thing to balance, the needs of other residents and the staff, and Don, too."

"I understand that," I sighed, paused, then added, "Don is sooo frustrated. He is an engineer, he is 64, he is used to feeling productive, being useful . . ."

"The disease affects everyone differently," suggested the activity director. "We have been trying everything. I mean — people in this room have agonized — ever since he got back from the hospital — the last time."

It wasn't until I actually typed that last sentence into this chapter, and began trying to make sense of the situation on paper, that I truly "zeroed in" on the activity director's words. They had "agonized" over how to help Don ever since he got back from the hospital . . . the last time?

That was in late September. The meeting with the social worker in January was the first time I had been told of such grave problems and deep concerns. I wished this same group had come to me earlier — included me in that agonizing — that I could have been part of a search for solutions before they decided there were no solutions.

I had continued to believe and trust that Wentworth's publicized training and experience with Alzheimer's disease would help them know how to work with Don. I knew there were many staff members who were "bending over backwards" to help him, and I was doing the same — trying to help them help him.

The occupational therapist's quiet words interrupted my thoughts.

"We appreciate what you said about Don's needing to — responding to feeling productive and useful," she said thoughtfully. "I think that is really a basic human need that stays with a person, no matter what. Maybe you can give us some direction, help us design some activities."

The activity director and the occupational therapist began to think out loud, to ask for my inputs. Was Don used to working at a desk? Did he have one at home? In response to my affirmative replies, we discussed the idea of bringing his desk to Wentworth. The three of us talked about what he used to do, what tools he worked with, what I might bring in or purchase — about what we could do to improve the situation for him.

Finally, we all paused . . . and it was quiet for a few moments.

I sat amidst the stillness thinking about the suggestion of bringing Don's desk to Wentworth. It was an excellent idea . . . but I couldn't help but wish it had been suggested earlier — or that I had thought of it myself months ago.

It was the social worker who broke the silence.

"We'll muddle through this," she said. "Hopefully it will not come to his having to go to another facility. We would really prefer it not to, as long as we can manage, or if we can start being able to manage what's being presented. Maybe some of these suggestions will help, or his condition will change and be more manageable and not be putting people at risk. That's the ideal. We really do care about Don. We all do."

And there, my tape ends.

I spent a great deal of time listening to that tape, typing the words into my computer, and poring over my notes, as I sought to tell this story fairly. What was really happening at Wentworth? What really was being said at this meeting? I still find it difficult to comprehend the whole situation, especially in view of how it continued to develop over the next few weeks . . .

Chapter Ten

I went from the meeting to Don's room. We had an extremely pleasant hour before dinner, and after we had eaten, I put a mellow tape into our cassette player. I urged him to stand, held him tightly, and in the tiny space in his room, we moved together, sort of "dancing" to the music. He seemed fairly alert, and was definitely responding to me — not with words, but with a big grin, an eagerness to cooperate, and an obvious sense of delight.

Later in the evening, the staff seemed extra busy, so I changed his diaper, washed his face and hands with warm water, and got him ready for bed by myself.

"I hate these," he muttered as I worked with the diaper.

"I'm sure you do . . . " was all I could think to say.

I found it challenging to comprehend our predicament there at Wentworth. Helping Don just didn't seem to be as difficult as they claimed. I knew I could not do so on a 24-hour basis, all by myself, at home. But when I helped out there at the nursing home, I didn't have much trouble. Why, I wondered, did they seem so insistent that the only solution was for me to move him out?

I walked into the nursing home lounge area a few days later, and noticed Don moving toward a female resident who was sitting in one of the chairs. I paused to watch. He had a big smile on his face, and was reaching out to touch and greet her, just as I had seen him do on other occasions. But this woman was seated, and looking down at her hands. Perhaps she would not see the warm smile on Don's face. Even if she did, perhaps she would feel vulnerable — if the staff was reflecting that this man was violent, there was no question that the residents would respond accordingly. I could envision exactly what was about to happen — and how the staff might react.

I hurried over, joined Don in greeting the lady, took his hand, and walked with him to his room.

On another occasion I found him alone in his room, just sitting in his chair. He had a rather puzzled look on his face, and was sort of mumbling to himself. I paused near the door, and listened.

"Didn't mean to . . . " he was saying slowly, over and over, sort of shaking his head in a sad and confused manner. Without even thinking, I knelt down beside him and asked what he meant — and of course, he couldn't tell me. I looked around for someone who might know what had happened, but no one was in sight.

I walked down the hall, checking other rooms as I went. They seemed to be short-staffed. When I finally located a new young aide, her almost curt response to my inquiry was, "Mr. Miller frightened a resident. The charge nurse filled out an 'incident' report."

As I walked back to Don's room, I thought about her words.

"How often," I wondered, "has some action of Don's been misunderstood or misinterpreted and termed 'aggressive' when it was simply frustration, or that kind and caring side of him reaching out to another human being?" There was no way to really know.

Several days after the meeting, the husband of a close friend helped me move Don's desk over to Wentworth. We placed it by the window in his room so that he could look out when he sat there. I brought a lamp, and some of his technical magazines that had lots of pictures. I brought pads of paper, various colored pens, and some of his old templates that I found at home. I purchased an abacus and a simple wooden puzzle.

Don responded positively to his new "office," and would sometimes sit at his desk busily "working" on various things.

Several of the staff members had been addressing Don as "Mr. Miller" all along. Sometimes when anyone approached him with that more formal, but very familiar greeting from his past, he would reach out and shake hands in his friendly, sincere manner. Now, if someone came into his room while he was at his desk and greeted him in that manner, he would often show him or her what he was "working on," perhaps even try to explain something about it.

During the next weeks, there were more times when things went well.

But, there were still occasions when Don's anger would surface. On Friday, February 11, 1994, my telephone rang a little after 8:00 in the morning.

It was the social worker at Wentworth.

"We are calling the Crisis Unit!"

I was there in 20 minutes.

So was the Crisis Unit.

I quickly assessed the scene. An ambulance was sitting in front of the entrance. Its back doors were wide open. A crowd from the facility had gathered. Don stood on the road, dressed in his nightshirt, chinos, and socks. Fortunately, the sun was shining, the weather was balmy, and the road was dry on that February morning!

The medics were urging him to step up into the ambulance. It was obvious he was refusing to do so.

I walked up to Don, looked him in the eye, smiled a greeting, and took his hand. I turned him away from that waiting vehicle, and quietly started walking with him back toward the front door of Wentworth.

"You won't be needing our services?" questioned the medics.

"No. We will not," I responded firmly, and as pleasantly as possible.

As we walked past the bystanders, two familiar faces held ill-disguised looks of anger. Many others held looks of understanding and quiet half-grins of approval.

A few days later, one of the L.P.N.s came to me quietly. She told me that after I "rescued" Don, they had all been told in no uncertain terms, to "Call Pat only after you have called the hospital, the ambulance is here, Don is on the gurney, and going out the door!"

On another day soon after, I called to see how Don was doing. Teresa answered the phone. "I don't want to be 'telling tales out of school,'" she said quietly, "but Bernice is on this afternoon and tonight, and things aren't going well."

Bernice . . . I suddenly remembered that a few weeks earlier, another loyal and concerned staff member on the unit had quietly given me an almost identical warning when I called — and concluded with a rather urgent sounding, "Come!"

On the surface Bernice seemed pleasant. But I had seen how she related to Don — had been told recently that she pushed him onto the bed, quickly put up the guard rail, and told him he had better stay there!

I understood Teresa's comment, and hurried over.

One evening, a young aide and I were leaving at the same time. He worked well with Don, and quietly shared that in his opinion some of the people on the day shift did not relate at all well to Don.

What all was happening, in regard to Don's care, on a one-on-one basis behind the scenes in this nursing home unit? No one but Don could know exactly, but I was getting a great deal of feedback that made me wonder if there were more negative things going on than I realized.

I finally began to accept that this situation was a losing one. It was stressful for me, and obviously for some of the aides assigned to care for Don. And it was surely no longer a healthy or comfortable environment for Don.

Sandy, Lisa, and I talked about the whole situation —

about the fact that Wentworth was saying that they could not handle Don.

As I reread Wentworth's brochures about their nursing home staff being trained in validation therapy, trained to care for people with Alzheimer's disease — thought about our careful decision to use Wentworth, and the whys behind that decision — I continued to wonder. Why couldn't they handle him? Why couldn't they help more people on their staff learn how to understand, respond to, and work with him?

Then, I remembered something. Long ago a good friend had commented, "We cannot cope with reality, if we cannot assess reality." It was a simple but powerful concept, and I realized there was good reason for the fact that it suddenly came into my mind.

In spite of the many people who cared deeply about Don, who knew how to help him, "reality" was that some people at Wentworth did not do well with him. And, "reality" was that the administrative people felt they had done all they could do, and that they really did not want Don in their facility.

Obviously I had continued to feel the situation could be worked on, changed, solved. The fact that things were not going to change began to truly "sink in." I had already talked with a few other nursing home administrators, but finally pulled out my old list of requirements and possibilities, and began to revisit facilities in earnest.

Been there. Done that . . .

And now, there was a new dimension.

Don had a "reputation" . . .

The people I spoke with in several facilities were cordial but firm. Wentworth was suggesting that we move Don out? If Wentworth couldn't "handle" Don, they were hesitant to say that they could.

A caring and obviously astute social worker at a fairly new facility — one I had not visited before — listened carefully to my story. When she asked why I was searching for a different nursing home, I told her that Wentworth considered Don violent and combative, that they could not handle him, and that they wanted me to move him out. I shared that I could work with him, and that they often called me to come over to calm him. When I questioned out loud, almost to myself, whether the reason I could work with him was that I was his wife, she shook her head.

"That is irrelevant," she said. "If you can work with your husband, others should be able to do so as well."

I agreed that there were some people who had no difficulty working with Don, but added that there were definitely those who did, and those who felt learning to help him was too challenging, and something they had no time for.

She shook her head again, this time a bit sadly.

"We have no openings at this point," she finally said slowly. She paused and appeared to be thinking, then added, "We might be able to admit your husband in several months. Perhaps you could find someplace that would take him on a temporary basis until we do have an opening."

I much appreciated her understanding and supportive attitude — but by that time I was convinced that I could not find a place that would provide that temporary situation. Even if I could find one, it seemed to me that making two more moves was just too much to do to Don — and too much for me to cope with at that point.

And, I knew that we could not make it at Wentworth for several more months while we waited for a possible opening.

On February 18, the social worker approached me in the hall.

"Don needs 24-hour-a-day care," she declared. It would cost an extra $10,000 a month. Would I like to "help?"

Ten thousand dollars more a month? Would I like to help!? I was struggling to pay the monthly cost as it was . . .

"No," said our lawyer.

Wentworth hired outside help. I had an opportunity to talk with the two women who arrived. They had been told that this man was violent and combative. They were each frightened by Wentworth's description, but both said they knew it would not be good for them to turn down an assignment because of fear. The one who worked the day shift was tall and well-built. She was told that she could "handle" a violent person. The woman who worked the evening shift shared that she was told she would be able to deal with such a challenge because she was "aggressive and feisty."

"He is such a nice man," they both said a few days after they started caring for Don. "We really love him . . . "

They began to share. They each were impressed by some of the staff members, especially the ones who seemed to like and do well with Don — those who were patient and kind. But there were others who were abrupt and impatient with him, who were too loud. Sometimes too many of them came in trying to control him — sometimes they were too rough. They noticed that every time there was any kind of problem, everyone was told to be sure to fill out an "incident" report.

I continued to look for, and at, other facilities . . .

On February 24, the social worker asked to see me in her office.

"We cannot handle Don," she informed me, continuing with the statement that I needed to transfer him — move him to another facility! Soon!

Her words caused the reality of our situation to truly sink in. Then several days later an incident occurred in regard to Don's care that incensed and deeply angered me, and I suddenly felt just as adamant as the administrative people.

They wanted me to move Don out, and I did not want him in their care!

At last, I heard about a facility in Vermont called The Phoenix Convalescent Center. It was a "progressive" place. The atmosphere was "homey." They had an Alzheimer's unit. The staff was trained to care for people with the disease.

Trained to care for people with Alzheimer's? My almost immediate reaction to the claim was one of skepticism. I had heard that before.

Then I caught myself. It was imperative that I approach this new possibility with a positive attitude, not with a cynical one.

The Phoenix was a long way from our home. It could be reached only on a narrow country road that wound its way through the mountains. But at that point, those things seemed irrelevant. Don's care was all that really mattered.

I called. I went over. I looked around carefully. I watched and listened. I asked many questions. I shared our situation with the woman who handled admissions. I liked her. My emotions were almost overwhelmed by her supportive, open-minded, and positive attitude.

With a handshake and a warm smile when I left, she said, "We will call you."

The call came the next day!

"We will take Don," said the friendly, yet efficient-sounding voice. "We think we can help him."

"Help him . . . "

Those almost unbelievably simple, but overwhelmingly welcome words brought tears to my eyes.

The move was set for March 7, 1994.

The administration people at Wentworth said they would be happy to provide transportation for Don, and an aide to ride along with him to assure that there were no "incidents."

Mike planned to pick up all of Don's things, and drive ahead of us to set up the new room.

When March 7 arrived, I found myself struggling with my emotions. Relief and hope, but also frustration and anger. I really did not want to encounter certain members of the staff. It would be too easy to say something I might regret.

I picked up the phone, and called Wentworth. Martha, our young R.N. friend, was on duty that morning. "Perhaps," I suggested, "I can meet you at the back door where the van will be waiting?"

She was by the door with Don when I arrived. Her eyes glistened with tears as she gave us each a hug and said "goodbye."

I found it sad to say "so long" to those people at Wentworth who had befriended and supported us, who had worked so hard at trying to help Don. But for me, there were no tears as I followed the van along the narrow, winding road. I was still dealing with other emotions. I was grateful to be on our way and out of that entire situation.

What lay ahead, I wondered. What would we find around the next bend in our road . . .

Chapter Eleven

There was plenty of time to think, to wonder, as I followed that van up and down the hills and around the curves along the two-lane country road. It was moving slowly and carefully, and the drive seemed to take forever. But the thoughts that drifted in and out of my consciousness seemed to be rambling and unrelated. I was tired. I felt numb as I mechanically drove along, matching the speed and moves of the driver ahead of me.

I had learned that Wentworth's compassionate driver, who had always been around to watch out for Don, took a personal day to drive his friend to Vermont in Wentworth's van! I was grateful for his presence there in the vehicle ahead of me. Even though Wentworth had provided an aide for the trip, I knew it would be that caring man who would be able to skillfully reassure Don if he became agitated or concerned.

Finally the van pulled into The Phoenix parking lot, and I followed closely behind. I eyed the community hospital, located on the other side of the large lot. There was a sense of *deja vu*. I couldn't help but think about the fact that Don had been taken to another hospital only four days after becoming a resident at Wentworth. I hoped we wouldn't be utilizing this one in the near future.

I found a space, parked the car, walked over to the van to meet Don and the others. They helped Don climb out, and all of us moved slowly toward the front door.

A second set of doors led into the unit where Don's room would be located, and was equipped with an alarm system similar to the one at Wentworth. As we walked through those doors, I watched two staff members cheerfully and gently reroute a wanderer. I had been impressed and hopeful when I first visited The Phoenix, and as the four of us walked in that morning, those same positive feelings surfaced. I felt an overwhelming sense that things would be better — that the atmosphere in this new facility would be different for us.

A wide, cheerful hallway led past several rooms, then opened into a combined nursing station and large lounge area. A huge skylight overhead, and big windows on each side of the room, gave the entire area an open and airy feel. On one side of the lounge were comfortable-looking chairs and couches, a television set, a piano, and a number of large and lush-looking potted plants. The opposite side of the room was filled with attractive tables and chairs for dining, chatting, or any activity for which that kind of setup was necessary.

An attractive gray-haired woman was playing the piano, and voices of both residents and staff joined together in singing some bouncy old and familiar melodies.

Amidst that jovial atmosphere, we stopped to check in at the desk. Then I thanked and bade "farewell" to Wentworth's driver and their aide. The R.N. in charge of the unit that morning greeted us warmly, signed Don in, and cheerfully led the way down the hall toward his new room.

Mike stood in the doorway with a welcoming grin. Once again, our loyal friend had done a marvelous job. There was no room for the desk, but Don's dresser, chair, and lamp were all in place. Our pictures were on the wall, and our TV/VCR and radio/cassette player were all hooked up! I set my picture and Don's photo album on the dresser beside the bed.

The room was tastefully decorated with subdued, but colorful, matching patterns in the curtains and spreads. The headboard and closets were made of warm-looking dark-brown wood. It looked cozy, even without our things, but those added pieces of our own definitely provided the finishing touch.

A whiff of fresh air drifted in through the slightly open window on that unusually balmy winter morning. The sun streamed in and filled the room, creating a bright and cheerful atmosphere.

Mike and I looked at one another with eyes of understanding, as he prepared to head back home. A new beginning. I knew we each hoped for good things.

Don's roommate, Ted, greeted us with a friendly smile. I soon learned that it was his wife, Dolores, who was doing such a wonderful job playing the piano.

Several staff members came in to greet and welcome us. The administrator who felt they could help, versus "handle" Don, stopped to say "hello" and see if there was anything we needed. A cheerful, friendly, vibrant woman, whose husband was in a nearby unit, came in to tell me they had an Alzheimer's support group. It would be meeting the next morning, if I felt I could make it.

At noon, an aide brought in trays that held a tasty lunch for each of us. After things had quieted down a bit, I carefully pulled the curtains part of the way around our little haven. Don readily stretched out on the bed, and I gratefully sank into our lounge chair beside him.

As the shifts changed, I watched "rounds" start. It struck me as a good idea that the two groups walked through the unit together, in and out of each room, as the preceding crew informed, alerted, and generally updated the new staff regarding the status of each resident. Cheerfully, warmly, sincerely, the entire group greeted us both.

I began to feel comfortable in the new surroundings. How I hoped the new situation would be a comfortable and more peaceful one for Don.

I stayed with him until he fell asleep that night, then headed for Victorian Manor, which was just a few blocks away.

I had spotted that beautiful old home when I first visited The Phoenix. "Bed and Breakfast in an Elegant Tradition," said their inviting-looking signpost. I knew I would not want to go all the way home the first night, and had decided it was exactly the environment I would need. As I guided the car out of The Phoenix parking lot, I was filled with a sense of relief, adventure, almost excitement. Our mission was accomplished. Don was settled in a facility that seemed to hold out new hope. How glad I was that I had made a reservation for myself at a special place.

I pulled up to the stately residence and just sat for a few minutes, taking in the inviting atmosphere of the big wrap-around porch and softly-lit windows. Moments later the gracious hostess ushered me up a winding staircase to the "Peach Room," a cozy room decorated in warm peach colors and filled with beautiful antique furniture.

The bed had a tall, ornate, hand-carved cherry headboard. A cherry washstand stood beside it with an open book full of signatures, addresses, and words of praise from previous guests. There was a huge bay window with neatly-draped crisp white curtains. I peeked into the large all-white bathroom. A bay window in that room was embellished with the same attractive curtains. A big white wicker chair with a high, hooded back sat near the window — a small matching table was carefully placed nearby. An old-fashioned, elegant-looking footed white tub sat in a corner.

I washed up, and soon made my way back down the broad spiral stairs to the spacious first floor. The immense, high-ceilinged, softly-lit library beckoned, with its plush-looking upholstered chairs and couches, a crackling fire, and the mellow sounds of classical music that filled the air.

It was a week night, and the room was empty. I was grateful for the quiet solitude, and eased into a large comfortable chair by the fire. Gradually my thoughts slowed and my body relaxed as I stared into the glowing embers, drifting along with the soothing strains of an orchestra's string section.

I was tired, but slowly a sense of peace began to fill my being. I knew the expense that was part of staying in those elegant surroundings would prohibit me from staying there on a regular basis. But for that one evening, it was perfect. It was important. It met a deep need . . . a need to do something special for myself.

I slept soundly in the comfortable queen-sized bed, and awakened refreshed the next morning. A new day. I wondered just what this new day would offer. I feasted on a sumptuous breakfast of grapefruit, bacon, eggs, and home-made raspberry muffins, sipped a steaming cup of hot herbal tea, took a deep breath — and plunged forward once again.

When I arrived at The Phoenix, I found Don up, just standing, in the new lounge area. His arms hung loosely at his sides. He looked so lost, but an eager look of recognition crossed his face as I drew near. I hugged him, gave him a kiss, carefully took our "skating position," and we went exploring.

We slowly made our way up and down the new hallways. Smiling, cheerful faces greeted us along every corridor, around every corner. There were alarms on double doors between units to protect wanderers. After checking with the staff about those alarms, I diligently followed their instructions and stopped them from ringing each time we went through a door.

There had been no openings in the separate Alzheimer's unit, and the administrator had decided to try Don in the more general section. I learned that the training that was supposed to help with Alzheimer's patients, was provided for all care givers at The Phoenix. The compassionate and knowledgeable approach behind the training started at the top, and seemed to work right on down to the cleaning staff and maintenance people. There was no question that the principles behind it made an enormous difference when it came to helping and working with any resident. I watched as many of the same basic techniques that I had learned worked well with Don, were successfully put into practice by the new staff.

The first month was difficult for Don. He simply stood, for long periods, with his arms just hanging at his sides — the same way I had found him on that first day. He did a great deal of sleeping. There were times when he became angry, and occasionally combative. The doctor who consulted at The Phoenix worked at readjusting medications, and the staff worked at getting to know and understand him. The more consistent, positive approach they took definitely appeared to lead to more consistent, positive responses and behaviors from Don, and soon the reports of anger on his part did not seem to be recurring as frequently. He didn't get "better" — the symptoms that accompany Alzheimer's and its downhill path did not disappear — but the trauma of the daily walk was certainly lessened.

Lisa came up from Virginia for a few days, and together we scoured the area for a more economical place for me to stay when I spent nights in Vermont. I planned to drive over at least twice a week, stay with Don that first day, spend the night, stay with him the next day, and drive home that night. We drove up and down the streets of the small community, checking out various options. I almost passed a bed and breakfast called the Picket Fence B&B, and it was Lisa who encouraged me to stop and check it out. The warm-hearted owner greeted us at the door and listened to our story. When she realized I would need a room two or three times a week, she said the rate would be only $25 a night! We had found exactly what I needed.

How good it was to see Lisa. It was wonderful to be together — great fun to do almost anything together! Just driving along the winding road from our house to The Phoenix, talking nonstop en route, was a delightful treat.

In spite of all the loyal friends who were keeping in touch, offering support, and letting me know they were there when

I needed them, I sorely missed our daughters. It was difficult to have them living so far away. Over those next few days, I thought again about how grateful I was for their cards, their calls, their visits — for the love of those two sensitive and thoughtful young women.

I was aware that the stress level had been overwhelmingly high over recent months, but I hadn't had time to notice that my fatigue was building. I was simply moving along step by step, almost automatically, trying to do what I knew I had to do.

Soon after Lisa left, I discovered just what a toll the situation was taking on me.

There had been a severe winter storm. I would get our driveway shoveled, come in to warm up, and several hours later find it covered with snow once again. The roads were treacherous, and I stayed home for three days. I kept in touch with the staff at The Phoenix, and several times had them bring Don to the phone so I could talk to him.

During the time I was home, I talked on the telephone with our lawyer about several things. She was upset about some papers I had signed at The Phoenix. She urged me to remember that once one signs some of their forms, a nursing home knows well how to use certain clauses against you for their own purposes, if its staff is so inclined. That is why some clauses are written the way they are.

I knew she was right. I felt defensive, but I knew that in reality I was angry at myself for not being more discerning, for being so trusting, especially after what we had just been through.

The morning I was finally able to head back to Vermont, I was struggling with many emotions, but glad to be on my way to see Don. Once I got past the traffic lights and congested areas, the road became less crowded. Although it was dry, there were places where the plow had left snow piled on the shoulders on either side, causing that country road to seem extra narrow. Several times I had a sense of feeling almost hypnotized, sort of staring and not seeing. I blinked my eyes and concentrated on clearing my vision. I drove along automatically, watching cars come toward me, then whiz by on the other side of the road. I sensed that I should find a place to pull over, yet thought, "No, I need to keep moving. I started later than I intended. Because of the storm, I haven't seen Don in three days. I need to get to him."

I veered to the left a bit. "Be careful," I thought, as I righted my course and continued along. Then suddenly, I was completely alert. The car was rapidly moving to the right, off the road over an area that was swept clear by the wind. I heard a long crunching and scraping sound, as I sought to right the car's movements. I found myself moving not only off the road, but onto a nearby field of snow. Although I had not been traveling with excessive speed on that winding road, it seemed as though it took a long time to slow the momentum of the car. As I looked ahead, a telephone pole lay precisely in front of the path in which I was moving. I worked to slow the car, to steer to the left, to miss that pole . . . Finally, the car came to a halt, just to the left, and just shy of that telephone pole.

I sat there . . . stunned . . . shaken. What if . . . what if I had veered to the left — into the pathway of a car coming toward me? What if I had swerved to the right at some other spot . . . and off a cliff, instead of into a field of snow? What if . . . ?

Fortunately, two men from the telephone company were working nearby, and saw what happened. They hurried over to check on me — then called for help from a garage with which they were familiar. A truck soon arrived to pull me back to the road. Now completely alert, I was on my way again. How lucky I was in so many ways. I had avoided a terrible accident. Help was immediate. I didn't hit the telephone pole. The right side of the car was badly scraped from the edges of a nearby metal road sign, but that was the extent of the damage. I sent up a prayer of thankfulness.

I shared the experience with David a few days later. He listened carefully, obviously taking in and comprehending the entire scenario. When I stopped talking, he simply looked at me for a moment or two, and then, with both compassion and concern, he said:

"Stress. Sleep deprived. Get some sleep . . . please . . . "

Not one word of condemnation. Not one ounce of blame. No "preaching" of any kind.

He knew that I knew what I needed to know.

I did.

Slowly, Don and I both settled into the new routine. Most of the people on this new staff were able to find the core of Don's true personality, and many of them developed very special relationships with him. They knew that when his anger did flare up, it was a symptom of the disease, and they helped reassure, calm, or divert him, rather than react.

Several of the men and women who worked on the unit seemed almost psychically connected. They worked together intuitively, creating a marvelous sense of teamwork. I could almost feel the deep caring and respect between them that radiated out to each of the residents. Watching them work together was an uplifting experience I have never forgotten, one that continues to fill me with great respect.

What a difference we can all make for one another! It is difficult to suffer losses, difficult to be in pain. And to me, it seems that feeling as though one is alone might be the most difficult of all. On the days when I was not with Don, it meant a great deal to me to know that there were others who cared about him, who would be there for him.

As the weeks went by, I was told all kinds of stories from those who worked with Don on a daily basis. We all enjoyed the times when his cheerful demeanor and delightful sense of humor surfaced.

One morning, I walked in the door at The Phoenix, and began looking around for Don. At first I didn't see him, then suddenly noticed two people way down at the end of the hall. As the pair moved slowly towards me, I realized it was Don, and a young aide named Joan. She was looking at Don as she chatted away, and the two of them began laughing as they approached, obviously having a marvelous time.

Then my gaze dropped down a bit, and I spotted Don's pants and diaper sitting dangerously low . . .

Joan noticed my glance, and caught my eye.

"I had a little trouble . . . " she chuckled, and she and Don exchanged cheerful grins.

As I looked at the two of them, I was filled with great respect for that outgoing and warm-hearted young woman. What a marvelous talent — to be able to transform what could have become a very difficult situation into one where Don was cheerful and content.

Another day when I walked into Don's room, he was up, dressed, and sitting in his lounge chair. He seemed to be in a good mood, and greeted me with a huge smile. Almost immediately, the activity director appeared, eager to report on the events of the previous day.

They had been playing "volleyball" in the lounge. The residents were seated in a circle — she was in the center, trying to get them to bat a balloon back and forth to one another. They were having great fun. Occasionally the balloon came Don's way. He would grab it, hold it, and grin! When she said, "Come on, Don, hit it to someone . . . " he would continue to just look at her, with that same mischievous grin. Did he really know what he was doing, she wondered? Whatever was going on in his mind, there was no question that he was enjoying himself, and it had "made her day," she said.

And then there was the time when I simply could not coerce Don into eating what was on his lunch tray. Finally, I suggested that we take a ride, as we had done on other occasions. On that particular day, I had a special plan in mind. Getting Don out to the car, into the car, out at a nearby supermarket, back in, out once again when we got to The Phoenix, and finally back to his room, was no small undertaking. But we returned with a special treat! I soon had fresh strawberries perched on top of dishes of ice cream from the little kitchen.

Now I had no problem enticing him to eat. There was no question about it. He knew what tasted good, as he happily accepted bites of the tasty combination, and with a silly grin on his face, even smacked his lips!

Along with the pleasant times when Don's sense of humor raised our spirits and charmed us all, there were times of seeming clarity that surprised us.

One morning, Doris, who often cleaned the rooms in Don's section of The Phoenix, quietly approached me. Some time ago, she said, she was working in Don's room. He was sitting in his chair. An aide had just finished helping him with lunch, and Doris noticed some particles of food lying on his leg. She approached Don slowly, caught his eye, mentioned her intentions, and gently brushed them off.

Don lunged forward. Was he going to grab her? She drew back in fear.

For the next week or so, Doris avoided getting too close to Don Miller. She carefully skirted around him when he was in the hall.

Gradually, she realized he seemed to be following her, or just standing and watching her, as she methodically moved along from room to room to clean. One day she gathered her courage, cautiously turned to face him, and smiled.

Slowly, haltingly, Don spoke.

"You . . . clean . . . " he said. "It's . . . okay." Tears slowly
trickled down his sincere face . . .

Tears quickly formed in Doris's eyes.

He had remembered!?

He felt bad?

He wanted to make amends?

It was a moment, she said, that she would never forget.

I knew I was spending a great deal of time with Don —
driving many, many miles back and forth from our home to the
nursing home. I was grateful that I had no other family responsibilities, no job commitment, and that I had the freedom and
time to be with him. But I was now more aware than ever that
I had to be careful not to get too tired — that I must pace
myself. Taking care of and being there for Don was vitally
important to me, but I had to remember I could not do that if
I didn't also take care of myself.

I continued to use my typewriter as a sounding board to
work through my emotions. There were still times when guilt
about not being able to keep Don at home hounded me. I
struggled with the idea that he was now physically so far away
from me — and even in another state. The idea that something
could happen, that he might die and that I might not be with
him, frightened me. I could see the disease advancing, and there
were times when the inevitable outcome threatened to completely unnerve me. How could I ever go on without him?

Fears of all kind plagued me. I had to keep reminding
myself that when there was no action I could take, the only
control I had was how I responded mentally to a situation. And,
reminding myself to take that one day at a time, to listen for
guidance, to choose positive thoughts and responses over
negative ones.

Even though intellectually I knew that each of these principles was vitally important, I found I had to work diligently to
put them into practice. I certainly did not always succeed, but

when I did, I seemed to understand them on a different level . . . and those experiences gave me hope — validated the idea that I could have some control over our situation. I could not change its reality, but I was learning that it was really true that choosing how I responded to each day, each challenge, made a huge difference in my own life.

I didn't have to be the second victim of this disease, or be at the mercy of guilt, fear, or any other negative emotions. On those rather rare, and often brief occasions, the realization was freeing — even exhilarating.

But, when the feelings of fear, anger, or depression seemed extra difficult to counter, I tried not to berate myself — to remember a comment David had once made — that there were times when it was important to "feel the feelings," to let them in, even if they were negative ones. I was grateful for close friends with whom I felt free to share my struggles, as well as my triumphs, and who felt comfortable sharing theirs with me. There were occasions when our senses of humor took over and we were able to actually laugh at ourselves — at the many challenges with which we each struggled.

One evening I called a long-time friend, and some of the negative thoughts and feelings that kept plaguing me came rolling out. My good and loyal friend listened patiently. When I had vented all my frustrations, and paused for breath, she quietly said:

"With all you have been dealing with — all you have been through — you deserve to be depressed!"

Just the right comment, delivered in just the right manner, at just the right moment! To her surprise, I burst into spontaneous, hearty laughter.

We were soon chuckling together, and able to move on to more positive thoughts.

"Perhaps the most important thing right now is the fight to survive," she suggested. "You are fighting. You are surviving.

You aren't going under. Maybe that's all that needs to happen right now."

What perceptive thoughts from a caring friend.

My trusty typewriter was giving me trouble. I wondered if perhaps it was time to join the "modern world," and change to a computer. I knew next to nothing about computers, and had no idea how to even determine just what to purchase. But with inputs from Lisa's husband, Bob, and other friends who were skilled in this "new to me" technology, I began to learn more, and my wondering soon turned to intrigue and enthusiasm.

Sometime in May, I got a phone call from Bob. He had found a Macintosh PowerBook at an unusually good price. "Macintosh computers are 'user friendly,' and I think this would be a perfect choice for you," he said.

"User friendly" was good! How tempting. We discussed it a bit further, and agreed that purchasing the one he had located was the thing to do.

I knew computers were shipped all the time, but it sounded like much more fun to go pick it up. And what a treat it would be to see Lisa and Bob! Did I dare take another quick trip?

"Yes," I decided.

I headed South.

Lisa and Bob had designed and built a lovely log home, high on a mountain outside their small college town. Visiting with the two of them, and spending two days at their cozy retreat, was delightful and refreshing. While they were at work, I sat on the warm and sunny deck listening to the silence, admiring the spectacular view, and practicing on my new computer.

We dined at a charming restaurant that had been created in a lovely old home. There were soft peppermint sticks in an old-fashioned candy jar by the front door — obviously a treat that others enjoyed as much as the three of us. The narrow hallways were filled with antiques, and around every corner there seemed to be another inviting little room. The tables were covered with red and white checkered tablecloths. Flickering candlelight added to the cozy atmosphere. We feasted on prime rib dinners, indulged in carrot cake for dessert, went to a movie, and Lisa and I talked late into the night. Coming home with my new acquisition was an added bonus.

I returned to discover that the days while I was gone had passed smoothly at The Phoenix. I was grateful — glad I had swallowed my fears and made the trip.

Late in June, Sandy and Katie flew up for two days. One day to see Don, we decided, one day for us. It was beautiful — warm, still, and sunny. Perfect for going up to a nearby lake. But there seemed to be too many obstacles to trying for a one-day outing at the lake with our neighbors' canoe. We looked at one another. Ah ha! Can't get to the lake to put the canoe in the water — we'll put water in the canoe!

Sandy and I relaxed in the sun that day, watching with delight as Katie enjoyed her very own, private "swimming hole."

Observing Sandy's happy three-year-old that afternoon was very different from the scenes of the following day. What a striking contrast it was to witness Katie's excitement and enthusiasm, to watch her growing, developing, learning on one day, and to spend the next day visiting Don in a nursing home.

When I took Sandy and Katie to the airport, I hugged and kissed them both, watched them get on the plane, watched that big plane taxi down the runway, take off, and disappear. My gaze came back to earth. The crowd at the gate was dispersing. I moved back down the corridor toward the exit. The couple in front of me walked hand in hand, obviously delighted to be with one another again. I thought of several other couples who had just boarded that plane together . . . and my thoughts and feelings were "off and running."

Never again. Never again would that warm smile greet me as either Don or I got off a plane, or that familiar hand hold mine as we started for home together. Never again would I travel with that handsome man dressed in his good-looking business suit and tie, wait for and board a plane together, head off for far-away places . . .

Those tears, so often perilously close to the surface, overflowed as I walked.

The days moved along . . . and the inevitable advancement of Alzheimer's continued. Don had more and more difficulty manipulating silverware. The dietary staff tried to include a variety of items that he could pick up as finger foods. There was always someone to help with meals, and how graciously they assisted with that elementary task. But in spite of everyone's sincere efforts, he was becoming less and less interested in eating. He continued to lose weight, and looked so thin and gaunt . . .

It was difficult to remember what he used to look like.

It was difficult to remember what he used to be like.

He began to spend more and more time just sitting. When he did insist on moving up and down the hall, he became tired quickly. That fatigue, combined with his deteriorating balance and unsteady gait, sometimes led to a fall. I was concerned, and so was the staff. Nevertheless, I found myself unprepared for the charge nurse's question one morning.

"Would it be all right if we occasionally restrain Don when he becomes overly tired?" she inquired hesitantly.

I just stood and looked at her for a moment. I knew restraints had occasionally been used at Wentworth and Brentwood, and it had bothered me. The idea of needing to use them now on a more regular basis — and having to okay, and hence condone, their use — was simply not something I was ready for. But at least she had asked me first . . . Finally, I found my voice.

"I much appreciate your asking me rather than just restraining him," I said slowly, still thinking about the question. "Let me think, and talk with you about it later."

Even though reports of Don's falling had became more frequent recently, the idea was not an easy one for me to consider. I struggled with her question as I watched and worked with him that day. I knew I could not always be there. I knew they could not always make the time to walk with him. I knew the request was truly in his best interest . . . and slowly began to realize I knew how I needed to respond.

The next morning the same young woman was on duty, and I stopped her in the hall when I arrived.

"It's all right to restrain Don if there are times when you feel you must, times when you feel you have no other choice," I said. Noticing the understanding and compassion in her eyes, I continued. "Thanks again for checking with me. We probably need to do that, but I do find it difficult to okay the idea . . ."

Because it was hard for Don to keep his balance, giving him a shower was becoming more difficult for everyone. It was Becky, one of his favorites and often his primary caregiver, who suddenly thought, "The bathtub!" Why couldn't they bathe Don in the large tub they used for some of the ladies? Would that be easier, or more of a challenge? To everyone's delight, the new approach was a great success. Becky shared that the first time they got Don into the tub, a wide grin of satisfaction appeared on his face as he slowly slipped down into the warm water.

Brushing Don's teeth, something that would ordinarily have been a simple process for him, was another challenge. He didn't seem to have the comprehension nor the ability to use a toothbrush, and the staff found it difficult to talk him into letting them brush them regularly. I had purchased an electric toothbrush, but he wanted no part of that noisy, vibrating tool.

One evening I was wielding his regular toothbrush, and watching Don's face as I worked. Suddenly, I realized I was hurting him. I stopped, and just stood there with his toothbrush in my hand. My eyes began to fill with tears.

Thoughts flashed through my head. The dental hygienist had said Don's gums were not in good shape, that it was vitally important for us to keep his teeth clean. But trying to do what needed to be done to prevent more serious problems was obviously painful for Don. That day I simply could not do it.

I stood looking at Don helplessly, and those tears began to roll slowly down my cheeks.

Suddenly Don reached up, cupped my chin with both of his hands, and looked into my eyes with a deep, caring look of love. No words were spoken. No words were necessary. His face and his eyes spoke volumes.

July 2, 1994, was Don's 65th birthday. I bought a helium birthday balloon, and made two lemon-jello sheet cakes to take to The Phoenix. When I arrived that morning, Don was sitting in a chair in the lounge, staring straight ahead. I set the cakes down, anchored the balloon underneath one of the pans, and went over to where he was sitting. I knelt down in front of him, looked into his eyes, and quietly said, "Happy Birthday."

I had surprised him, which might have been all right under normal circumstances, but how bad I felt as I watched those familiar eyes fill with tears, and those tears slowly roll down his cheeks.

Gradually the tears were replaced with a grin, but it was definitely not the best of days. We shared the cake. He responded to the caring good wishes from everyone — but he was soon grimly moving up and down the hall, gripping my hand as he went. I finally succeeded in getting him to sit in his chair and jokingly curled up on his lap to keep him there. Slowly his mood improved, and when I finally left that evening, he was asleep, once again with that half-grin spreading over his face.

"But what a sad way to spend a birthday," I thought, as I drove to the Picket Fence that night, struggling to see the road through the blur of tears . . .

What a relaxing retreat the nights at that bed and breakfast always were. Sometimes I would fix a hot cup of tea in the little dining room when I arrived, and on occasion, chat with the friendly and caring owner. The rooms were small and the surroundings very simple, but I always felt a sense of warmth and welcome there.

One morning in August, I walked into Don's unit just before lunch, and discovered that he was very agitated. He had been pacing up and down the halls all morning, and had rebuffed everyone's attempts to talk him into sitting down.

In spite of my added efforts, and the staff's cheerful support, he remained restless and irritable. I was able to talk him into stopping for lunch, but as soon as he finished, he insisted on being on his way again. So, we walked the halls together.

The evening was just as difficult as the day had been. One of the aides helped me get him into his nightshirt and ready for bed, but he did not want to lie down. He sat on the edge of the bed and glared at the world.

I stood there looking at his knitted brow, and the familiar face that was so full of frustration, and wondered how to help.

Suddenly I remembered the small pink plastic basin I had stashed away in his cupboard — just large enough for me to fill with water and still carry without spilling the contents — and just large enough to soak Don's feet. "Perhaps the next best thing to a warm bath before bed," I had thought when I purchased it.

Soon I was kneeling on the floor, massaging Don's feet in the warm water.

The room was quiet.

Don continued to glare. I was caught up in my own thoughts.

I glanced up, and noticed that his scowl seemed a little less intense, his face a bit more relaxed.

"Good . . ." I thought.

The warmth of the water on my hands began to relax me as well.

The sound broke my reverie.

"Nice . . ."

I looked up, and found Don's eyes fixed on my face, his gaze intense.

We looked into one another's eyes.

His began to light up with apparent excitement, delight, joy . . . and a wide grin spread slowly across his face. He took both of his hands and grasped my shoulders . . . in almost an embrace . . . looked deep into my eyes . . . and suddenly exclaimed:

"It's you!"

My heartfelt words responded to his. "It's me . . ."

A moment that defies description.

He continued to watch every move I made with a contented, happy look. I dried off his feet, dusted them with bath powder, got him settled in bed, and cleaned things up. I finished, moved over to the bed, lay down beside him, and put my left arm across his chest. He moved over a bit, and gently patted my arm. We lay there next to one another on that narrow hospital bed, in that nursing home so far from home . . . together . . . in the deepest sense of the word . . . for those few moments in time.

Chapter Twelve

All the way home I thought about those moments, and about some of the other times when Don's love for me had broken through the wall of Alzheimer's disease. Those cherished memories often brought tears to my eyes, but, oh, how they warmed my heart.

Yet I sensed that somehow if I was going to survive, going to be able to walk on, I needed to be realistic. I must not romanticize, or fantasize, about the past. Our love wasn't perfect. Our relationship was not a "storybook" one. We had had our share of difficult and challenging times before Don's illness.

But the bottom line was that our love had grown, changed, sustained us, and provided deeper meaning than I could ever have imagined. It was surviving, and even triumphing over, the stresses in our lives, and I was deeply grateful.

I arrived at our house, walked in the front door . . . and abruptly became very aware of my home's appearance.

As usual, the living room was fairly neat, but everywhere else there were piles of paper and miscellaneous items — the same piles that had been there when I left. Some of them had been there for many weeks . . . And not only were the usual items on the kitchen table and kitchen counter, but now there were even things scattered all over the dining room table! An almost overwhelming sight. Suddenly all of my philosophical thoughts vanished.

There were so many thing that needed attention. And every time I took care of one thing, it seemed as though two more appeared.

I just stood, looking at the mess. I half considered at least paying a few bills, then decided, "No." It was late. It was time to quit. I would deal with paperwork some other day. For now, I would send my love to Don, and give a prayer of thanks for the moments we had just shared.

The temperature, as well as the calendar, reflected that fall was approaching. As the change in the weather became increasingly noticeable, I changed from lighter clothes to jeans and warm sweatshirts.

The gradual changes in Don were equally noticeable. He spent more time than ever just sitting. His need to keep moving seemed less strong, and his ability to do so was obviously deteriorating. He slept a great deal during the day. Often he would still be in bed or asleep in his chair when I arrived at 10:00 or 11:00 in the morning. He showed less initiative as far as picking up finger food, and less interest in anything we offered. There were times when he simply would not eat. When that was the case, I tried feeding him. Occasionally, he would nod, and begin to doze off in the middle of a meal.

The days and weeks began to blend into one another. As I drove back and forth on those winding roads that fall, I watched the trees turn to spectacular colors. Viewing the breathtaking mountainsides filled me with a sense of awe — a sense of order and purpose — a sense of being part of something greater than myself. There were deep reds and bright reds — oranges, golds, and yellows. The dark green of nearby pine trees created a striking contrast, and the mountains and rolling countryside became a gloriously beautiful panorama. The narrow little road was often a busy one, with "leaf peepers" now replacing the summer vacationers.

Don's roommate, Ted, died that fall. I would miss his cheerful smile . . . His wife and family were by his side, and I was glad. I didn't like the idea of anyone dying alone.

We moved Don's bed and all of his things to the other side of the room. It was nice to be closer to the window, to the sunlight when it streamed in, to have an opportunity to open that window if the room got too warm.

I don't think Don had any awareness of the move or the reason for the change, but I surely did. For several days, the empty bed sat there. It was a constant reminder. One day Don's bed, too, would be empty . . .

I kept checking my emotions, checking my thoughts, working on my head. It was good to be aware of realities, but I knew I must not dwell on them.

Before long, a handsome gray-haired gentleman became Don's new roommate. Warren had had a stroke, but his good humor and warm-hearted smile were very much intact. His wife was not living, but a young man appeared on a regular basis. One day I asked that young man — was he Warren's son?

"No, just a friend and neighbor," was his quiet response. "*Just* a friend and neighbor . . ."

What a very special "friend and neighbor."

October of 1994, Sandy's second daughter, Christina Ann, arrived. My thoughts vacillated back and forth, as I struggled with my desires, my priorities, and my fears. I wanted to go to Raleigh to meet the newest member of our family, and I wanted to stay at home so I could spend time with Don. But Christy would not be brand new for long. On the other hand, Don did not look good to me . . . What if something happened while I was gone?

I tried to reassure myself — struggled to sort out my feelings — to calm the what-ifs. I knew I should not allow fear to govern my decisions. All had been well when I returned from Lisa and Bob's . . . I decided that I should go.

I was gone for only three days, but as I discovered on earlier trips, that brief visit was a valuable break for me. Late one night, Sandy and I curled up on the bed and shared thoughts and feelings about birth, about life, about death, about love. Katie warmed my heart with hugs and grins and giggles, and it was good for my soul to hold new little Christy in my arms.

When I arrived back at The Phoenix after that visit, it was about 10:00 in the morning. Don was still in bed, still in his nightshirt. The head of the bed was raised, and he was sitting up. His tray stood beside his bed. Ensure was all over him, on the bed, and on the floor. Crumbs and pieces of food lay on the covers. His hair was a mess, and I soon discovered he was very wet.

But he grinned at me when I walked in the door! Almost a devilish grin!

Becky was his primary care giver that day. She and Alicia, another one of Don's favorites, saw me arrive and promptly followed me into the room. Don had been giving them a terrible time. He would not eat. He would not get up. He would not cooperate with anyone! He had been taking a donut apart and throwing pieces at a new girl!

Finally, Becky had said, "If you don't stop, I'm not going to come in here anymore!"

Don had stopped! But he wouldn't let them clean him up.

With my arrival, he quite cheerfully let Becky and me work our way through the debris, get him cleaned up and ready for the day. He truly seemed rather satisfied with himself! That special "boyish" sense of humor of his could definitely surface now and then. Throughout the morning, I had to chuckle every time I thought of the almost comical scene.

Alicia shared that while I was gone, it had required three of them to take care of Don one morning. When they finally finished, he stormed out of the room, stumbling as he went, and started down the hall. She had followed to make sure he didn't fall. When he saw her, he glowered at her. Then, with just the hint of a grin, he reached toward her in a menacing way, as if he were about to attack her.

She laughed and said, "I'm not afraid of you!"

Don had laughed with her, and they continued down the hall together.

What an understanding, sensitive, and enlightened response on Alicia's part. How easily someone could have responded differently . . . and received a very different reaction from Don.

Gradually, the colorful leaves that had decorated the Vermont countryside over the last month fell to the ground, leaving the hills and valleys looking gray and barren. It was easy for my thoughts to turn gray and barren as well.

I wanted to be with Don, but it was increasingly difficult to know what to do during our time together. I packed a small carrying case with tapes filled with cheerful, lively music to play in the car, and brought a new supply for Don's room. I made cookies to munch as I drove, and packed some to share with Don and the staff. I brought two simple and lighthearted A. A. Milne books of poems that he used to read to the girls, and his book of poems from college to read to him, hoping to lift both of our spirits.

As I left for Vermont one morning, I decided to stop at our neighborhood jewelry store to get a battery for my wristwatch. While I waited at the counter for the man to put it in, my eyes scanned the items in the display case. A small gold outline of a heart that had a pearl set in the middle caught my eye. It was so pretty! As I stood admiring it, I realized that the small pearl in the center of the heart was what appealed to me.

It took a moment, and then I knew why. The attraction was connected to a scene in a movie Don and I had seen long ago, called "David and Lisa."

We had both enjoyed the heart-warming and beautifully told story about two disturbed young teenagers, David and Lisa. They meet in a psychiatric hospital, and the scene I remembered shows the two of them walking in the hospital gardens. Lisa, who struggles with her identity and always has to speak, and be spoken to, in rhyme, says to David, "David, David, what do you see?"

With a warm and caring smile, David responds, "I see a girl, a pearl of a girl."

A pearl.

"A pearl of a girl" was the connection, and it had become transposed in my mind to "a pearl of a guy."

Don Miller was a pearl of a guy!

I walked out of the store with a fresh battery in my watch, and a tiny gold heart, now placed on a long gold chain — a simple piece of jewelry that became a cherished possession as soon as I placed it around my neck.

That afternoon, I encouraged Don to sit in his chair, then I sat on his lap. I showed him my wonderful new necklace, reminded him about the movie, about that special scene, told him he was a "pearl of a guy" — and that he would be in my heart forever.

He appeared to be listening carefully, and reached out to touch the tiny heart. Then he took it between his thumb and fingers, and gently caressed it .

I continued to stay overnight several times each week. On one trip to Vermont, I learned that the owner of the Picket Fence had decided to utilize her rooms as an adult home. So one cold and dismal afternoon, I went looking for a new place to stay. When I walked into the entrance of the Fireside Motel, and spotted the glowing fireplace in their small but inviting-looking lobby, I knew I had found the spot for which I was searching. And, it was even closer to the nursing home.

The temperature continued to drop, and the countryside was soon white with snow. Winter had arrived a bit early in the Northeast. When I headed for home late at night, the roads were often treacherous. As I drove along the dark roads in the sparsely populated areas, with only occasional lights from a passing vehicle, I was especially grateful for my cell phone.

With the colder weather, as well as shorter and often darker days, my struggles with depression intensified. David asked questions. How was I feeling, focusing, concentrating? Was I forgetting things? How was I sleeping . . . and eating . . .

"You have done everything possible," he said quietly. "There is no more action to take — no way to fight, nothing more you can do for Don, other than walk the road with him. It's easier for the feelings to take over now."

"Definitely a true fact," I thought. My recent struggles to keep negative emotions at bay were a perfect example.

He was watching, he had said, to make sure that walking this road did not take too great a toll on me. I was grateful that he was watching.

I had a deep desire to survive, not only physically, but also mentally. In spite of all of my sincere efforts, I found myself struggling with depression. Winter was upon us — a time of year when it was often more difficult to stay healthy even under normal conditions. I was well aware that for me, these were definitely not "normal" conditions. I was tired. And I had a cold.

I had moved slowly off the Zoloft soon after Don arrived at The Phoenix. Things had been going well, and I didn't really like using an antidepressant. But now, both David and I agreed that it would be worth trying a low dose once again. The antidepressant might not only help me maintain my emotional stability, but that stability might also help my immune system function more efficiently.

The day before Thanksgiving, Mark, a contractor who had also become a special friend over the years, was doing some work at the house for me. When he left that day, he gave me a hug.

"My wish for you for Thanksgiving," he said, "is that Don gets a 'window' so that you can have some special time together."

What an awesome comment . . . Obviously I had been sharing more than I realized. And Mark had been listening with his heart. A "window" of clarity . . . where Don might know me . . .

I knew what he meant.

And how much his thoughtful words and compassionate wish meant to me that night.

I awakened the next morning to a cold, but clear and sunny, Thanksgiving Day. As I headed for Vermont and into the higher elevations, the frost on the trees glistened in the early morning sunlight. The sky was blue. The roads were dry. It was an absolutely gorgeous day.

In spite of the circumstances in which Don and I found ourselves, I breathed a prayer of thanks for the love between us, for all that was good in our lives, for the fact that he was in a place where people cared about him . . . and where he was receiving the best of care.

When I walked through the front door of The Phoenix, I was greeted by the familiar aroma of turkey and dressing. The walls along the corridor were decorated with colorful hand-made Thanksgiving decorations. Cheerful greetings warmed my heart.

Becky and Alicia were sitting with Don at a table in the lounge. Alicia quickly found a plateful of the traditional treats for me, and I sat down to join them.

As Alicia helped Don with dinner, Becky confided quietly. "Don was in tears all morning. I told him that Pat was coming. That comment always helps calm him down — or cheer him up."

Even before Thanksgiving was over, there seemed to be signs of the approaching Christmas holiday everywhere I looked. I found it difficult to get enthusiastic about the season, but for Don's sake — and for my own — I knew I would try.

In the past, Don and I had almost always found a place to cut down our own tree, and the wonderful pine aroma that filled the house was very much a part of our Christmas. But when he was no longer at home, I hunted for two small artificial Christmas trees — one for Don, and one for me. I decorated them both with tiny green lights and little red hearts, and each year re-covered them with drops of pine-smelling oil.

I took Don's tree to The Phoenix, and set mine up at home. I baked batch after batch of his favorite Russian Tea Cakes, filled a big cookie tin to have in his room, and placed mounds of cookies on separate plates for the staff. I bought him a big box of the milk chocolate buttercreams that we both always enjoyed.

I found my spirits lifting, and realized my efforts to make Christmas for Don really were helping me as well. I purchased cards, spent my free afternoons and evenings writing notes on them, and sent them on their way.

I began to find caring greetings from friends both near and far in our mailbox, many of them filled with words of hope and encouragement. Occasionally that sense of a Presence, a sense of peace that had seemed to elude me in recent months, crept into my being. Perhaps the Zoloft was helping. Whatever was involved, I began to find it easier to keep my thoughts and emotions focused on the positives.

I stayed home that Christmas Eve and curled up in my favorite chair with a book. The crackling fire, the little Christmas tree, the familiar music, all added to my uplifted spirits. Thoughtful telephone calls from each of the girls added the finishing touch to that traditional "family" night. I was alone — but I didn't feel lonely. Early the next morning, I headed for Vermont to be with Don.

How hard the staff worked at making each holiday a cheerful occasion. There were always decorations of all kinds on the walls, the tables, the counters of the nursing station, and on blouses and shirts and heads. Their friendly smiles and good-natured greetings to visitors and residents alike, added to the warm environment.

When I arrived at the nursing home, I found Don seated in the lounge area. He had a big red Christmas bow carefully pinned on his shirt, and a small object clutched in his hand. A little later, Alicia quietly told me its story.

"We found a little porcelain frame in the shape of a wreath," she explained. "We got it for Don, and found a picture of you to fit inside. I hope you don't mind that we cut it up . . .

"When we gave it to him this morning, he cried," she told me. "And he has been clutching it in his hand ever since," she added softly.

When we moved back to his room, there were more presents. I found a number of small elegantly-wrapped packages under his little tree, and special cards from several members of the staff. There was even a card for me from Don. Becky had carefully searched for a special one and signed it for him. A small stuffed Christmas reindeer hung from his lamp, with a tag that said it was from Doris, the friend who kept Don's room so very clean. There was a Christmas stocking filled with candy and accompanied by a lovely card with good wishes from the entire staff.

What thoughtful gestures from those kindhearted people!

I lit the lights on our little tree, put a Christmas tape into the cassette player, and shared my surprises with Don.

In spite of the fact that our Christmas was being celebrated in a nursing home, in spite of the sad reality of the disease that stalked Don, somehow that special spirit of Christmas returned, crept into the room, and into my heart.

But there can be times when it is difficult to retain the Christmas spirit . . .

At a holiday luncheon a few days later, an acquaintance bluntly and rather abruptly asked me, "Do you go to see Don so often for you or for him?"

I was caught off guard. I could hardly believe what I'd heard. In spite of my vow to do this my way and not be affected by other people's opinions, anger and defensiveness began to well up. Whose business was it but mine? And what difference did it make to her?

I paused, not wanting to say something I would regret. Finally, I responded.

"For me, I guess. Perhaps he does not always know who I really am, but I know who he is. And I will always remember that I was there."

The answer seemed to satisfy her, and the conversation between the group of women moved on to other topics.

But her question continued to bother and anger me. I hadn't realized how vulnerable I really was. How very easy it is for each of us to make a simple unthinking remark that hurts another person. I know there have been times when I have done it myself — times when I regretted some comment I made, and probably times when I was completely unaware that I had hurt or upset someone.

That evening, I sat at my computer trying to sort out my thoughts and feelings. I tapped away on the keys, and looked at the words that appeared on the screen.

Perhaps I went for Don, and for me. I really knew my visits were important for both of us. On the other hand, maybe I should give myself a break, go a little less often, perhaps not stay overnight every time.

But it did seem as though the staff had more trouble when I didn't turn up regularly . . . And I missed Don. I wanted to spend time with him . . . even if he was very different from the person he used to be . . . even if he did not know exactly who I was much of the time.

Late one morning a few days later, I was trying to decide whether to respond to some special Christmas notes, pay some bills and balance my checkbook, or go to see Don. I seemed to be having a difficult time making a decision. The conflict of emotions was strong.

"Go. Don't go.

"You should. You shouldn't.

"I want to. But I should stay here and try to dig my way out from under some of this paper."

Finally, my urge to see Don became stronger than my desire to stay home. "Go," my head seemed to say. "Be with Don. One day he won't be there to be with . . ."

I was soon driving the familiar mountain road.

When I walked in the door of Don's unit, Tom was standing nearby, passing out medications to the residents. That warmhearted and skilled LPN was married, had two young children, and was studying to become a Physician Assistant in his "spare" time! Tom was always especially good with Don, and deeply concerned about his welfare. That morning, he greeted me with an obvious sense of relief and welcome, and immediately said, "Don has been in tears. Things have been going from bad to worse, and no one has been able to work with him or calm him down. I'm awfully glad to see you . . ."

My eyes followed his gaze.

Don sat in the main lounge, restrained in a chair, crying.

What if I hadn't come . . .

I hurried over, knelt in front of him, and looked into those familiar blue eyes . . . eyes that were overflowing with tears of obvious frustration and sadness.

Slowly his eyes focused on my face, then met mine. As I reached out to wrap my arms around him, his reached back, clutched me . . . then clung to me. Instead of just tears, his body began to shake with deeper and deeper sobs of emotion.

I held Don's shaking body, struggling to control my own emotions. "Sobbing one's heart out," was a phrase I had heard expressed . . . At that moment I truly understood its meaning.

Slowly his sobs began to subside. I carefully felt for the restraining belt, undid it, and helped him stand. I hugged him, held him close to me there in the middle of the sea of faces — some blank, some filled with great compassion.

I gently positioned our arms in the now familiar "skating position," cautiously helped Don walk across the lounge, and slowly we made our way down the hallway to his room. I helped him sit down in his chair, carefully settled myself on his lap, and wrapped my arms around him once again.

We just sat. I stroked his hair, kissed his wet cheek, laid mine on his.

After a while, I eased myself off Don's lap, went over to the sink, ran the water until it was warm, soaked a washcloth, wrung it out, and carefully wiped his face. Gradually he began to relax. I shaved him, combed his hair, and sat back down on his lap.

I gave him a hug, a kiss — pulled back to look him in the face again — and, through my tears, smiled at Don.

As I looked at the transformation, I thought, "Yes, I need to follow my own inner voice — my own sense of guidance.

"Why do I go to see Don so often? Because I want to. And this is why." Was it for me or for Don? In the very depths of my being, I knew the answer. I did come for both of us.

I stayed a long time that evening, curled up on the hospital bed next to Don, waiting to make sure that he was asleep before I left. As I walked down the hall on my way out, my eyes filled, and tears began to trickle down my face.

Tom had worked a double shift, was still there, and working at the desk when I walked by. As I told him "goodnight," he looked at me closely.

Then, with both empathy and concern reflected in his voice, he quietly said, "Drive carefully . . ."

Chapter Thirteen

New Year's morning 1995 dawned cold and overcast, with big fluffy snowflakes slowly drifting down from the sky. I checked the roads. Not bad. I bundled up and was soon on my way to be with Don. The snow began to fall in earnest as I moved into the higher elevations. As visibility diminished, I drove along more slowly. I finally pulled into The Phoenix parking lot, carefully slipped the car into an open slot, zipped up my jacket and pulled on my gloves to weather the cold and continuing flurries, and hurried toward the front entrance.

The first thing I saw, as the automatic doors swung open, was a huge poster that said, "Happy New Year!" The cheerful sign was hand painted by the staff, and provided a warm welcome on a very cold day. I stomped the snow off my boots and hurried down the hall, returning greetings or smiling at the familiar faces there, keeping an eye out for that special guy of mine. He might not have looked like my "special guy" at that point, but if I worked hard at looking past what my eyes saw, I could always find him.

No Don standing near the door. No Don sitting in the lounge. As I moved on, I didn't see his familiar form moving slowly along the railings in the hall. A voice behind me said, "Hi, Pat. Don hasn't been feeling very well and is in his room." I turned to thank Alicia, hurried along and into Don's room.

As I moved past the first bed, I returned Warren's big grin and cheerful "hello." From behind the curtain partition appeared Don's brown recliner, our pictures on the wall of Don and the girls, and his photograph of the sunset across the lake.

Then I saw our floor lamp and the tiny Christmas tree with its twinkling green lights. As I moved around the curtain, I found the one for whom I was looking.

He was asleep. He looked so peaceful. I took off my jacket and gloves and exchanged my snowy boots for the slippers I kept there. After settling into the chair next to his bed, I carefully slipped my hand around the limp one that lay on the covers. A flicker of his eyes and half a grin told me my presence was noticed.

I soon learned that Don had been in bed all morning, that he had a slight temperature and flu-like symptoms. I was well aware that winter months could be difficult ones for people in nursing homes, and during the last few weeks, a number of the residents at The Phoenix had been ill with the flu.

I had not intended to stay overnight, but as the day progressed and Don remained in bed, I was hesitant to go all the way home. I called the Fireside, and then other motel and bed and breakfast spots I had used before. I quickly became aware that New Year's Day — which also happened to fall on a Sunday — was no time to be trying for accommodations for the night.

Finally, I checked with the staff, then lay down on the bed next to Don. Soon he was asleep, and gradually I fell asleep right beside him — backed up against the railing on the bed to keep from landing on the floor. Metal railings are not the softest, and hospital beds are not the widest, but it was nice to feel his body next to mine as I drifted off. It had been a long time since we had spent the night together. It seemed to me that perhaps Don, too, sensed the closeness, the "rightness."

Those "windows" continued to appear — times when there seemed to be a bit of clarity — times when I felt so strongly that somewhere in the depths of his being, Don recognized me. There also continued to be those infrequent and isolated occasions when a comment rolled out that was so very full of meaning. It was just in December that a young aide told me she had jokingly asked Don to give her a kiss on the cheek, and that his response had been, "No," that he was a "one-woman man!"

Such a special, loyal, and loving person he was. It amazed me that at that point amidst this devastating disease, he had such a thought and was able to express it.

I was trying to make myself presentable in the little bathroom connected with Don's room the next morning, when I heard Becky talking with someone outside the door. I recognized the second voice, couldn't quite place it, then realized it was the doctor who covered the nursing home. "He must be doing his early morning rounds," I thought to myself. I wanted to talk with him, but as I peered into the mirror, I was definitely not impressed with the image that stared back at me. I wasn't quite prepared for much of anything at that point, but did the best I could with a flick of my comb, and went out to greet him.

I watched as he checked Don's lungs, listened to his heart, and generally assessed the situation. When he finished, I walked out into the hall with him. We briefly discussed his findings, and I repeated the thoughts we had discussed earlier regarding Don's care — about not treating any illness if he got sick — about not sending him to the hospital. We all knew that we could not solve the underlying problem, and he assured me that he remembered how we felt. He would make sure that everyone on the staff was aware of our wishes. I sensed compassion and understanding in his eyes, his voice, his entire approach.

I spent the second day of January with Don. That evening he still had a slight temperature, but seemed to be comfortable. Should I head for home? No, I decided, I would stay in Vermont, if I could find a spot. I called the Fireside again. The cozy little room that was set back behind the others, one that I had used many times before, sounded extremely inviting.

I was delighted to find that it was now available. And I was grateful for my airline carry-on bag, which was sitting in the back of the car. I had packed a few extra items in it when I first started driving to Vermont, thinking that bad weather or road conditions might occasionally make getting home when I planned impossible. What a "lifesaver" it turned out to be that night, and many evenings in the days ahead.

It was very late when I picked up the key from a box by the motel office, and let myself into the room. What a marvelous treat it was to stretch out across the luxurious expanse of that queen-sized bed in such attractive surroundings.

The next morning Don's temperature was up. By early afternoon it had risen to 103 degrees, and by early evening we discovered it had hit 104.9! I quickly agreed that we should use Tylenol in an attempt to lower it and keep him comfortable.

It didn't take long for the thermometer to register a lower temperature, but for me, leaving Don was out of the question. I stayed put, this time stretched out, sort of, on the lounge chair beside the bed. The night staff moved silently in and out of the room. They always seemed to notice when I was awake, and their hushed greetings were warm and caring.

A few hours later, I realized that Don wasn't asleep. He seemed to be sort of "searching" with his eyes and facial expression. I moved from the chair, eased myself onto the bed beside him, and sat watching his face — wondering what was going on in his mind. I was leaning on my arm, and sat back a bit to get into a more comfortable position. When I did that, a thin shaft of light from the parking lot that came through the small break in the curtains, fell squarely on his face, and in his eyes. I sat back up to shield him.

Suddenly, my mind was filled with thoughts.

That small beam of light that I had blocked . . . It came from a source beyond the room, and that source was much greater than the little bit of light in the room. There must be a Light, a Love, beyond our love, that is the source of, and greater than, our love. Our love was part of that greater Love, just as the dim light in the room was part of that greater light beyond the room.

I'm sure I had read ideas along these lines in other people's writings, and similar thoughts had crossed my mind before . . . but at that moment the sense of their reality completely filled my being.

As I sat there beside Don, thinking about the sad downhill path he was walking, his condition over the last years, and the bleakness of his future, I was filled with an overwhelming sense of love for him. And I knew he loved me deeply. I did not want to part.

Yet in those moments, there was no question in my mind. In spite of the love I knew we had for one another, there is that even greater Love that we are all a part of . . . and I wanted Don to know that if he saw or sensed such a Love, it was all right to move on toward it . . . that it would not diminish, nor would we lose, the love between us.

So I shared . . . and shared.

There was no real indication that he could hear me, but somehow I felt that on some level, he did . . . that he might be able to comprehend something of what I was saying. Gradually, his eyes began to close. I carefully moved back to the lounge chair, and soon drifted off to sleep.

Ever since I had arrived on New Year's Day, Don had been in bed. We worked at turning him and changing his position. By January 5, his temperature seemed to stay between 102 and 103 degrees. They discovered that his oxygen count was low, and the staff continued to monitor it.

I kept offering food, but over the last five days, he had eaten very little. For some time, we had been using Ensure to supplement or replace meals. Now he would not pull from the straw, and often just let the liquid roll out of his mouth when we tried using a cup. He would take a fair amount of crushed ice and a few sips of water.

As I sat beside the bed that evening, I began to realize that his breathing had become extremely erratic. Suddenly, he didn't appear to be breathing at all! He looked terribly still. Could he have died? I felt a wild pounding in my heart. Hardly even thinking, I shook him gently to see if he would awaken.

Don opened his eyes, glared angrily at me, then closed them again, and appeared to stop breathing.

With growing panic, I ran out to the hall.

Tom stood by his medicine cart just a few doors away.

"Please come!" I called.

Struggling to keep my emotions under control, I tried to tell him what had happened as the two of us hurried back into Don's room.

"What if that is the last look between us!" erupted, as I voiced the thought I hardly dared consider.

Tom quickly checked Don's vital signs.

"He's okay, Pat," he reassured me, then patiently explained that Don's breathing pattern was a form of periodic "non-breathing," called Cheyne-Stokes Respiration. Then with a grin that reflected both compassion and support, he added, "You'd better get comfortable in that chair, girl."

I did just that — feeling completely drained, but over-whelmed with relief.

I was there.

I was with Don.

But I didn't want our walk to end that way.

I had been with Don at The Phoenix for almost a week. I was tired. My neck hurt. My eyes were scratchy and burning as I faced another new day. "But no matter," I thought. "This is where I want to be."

As I moved from one moment to the next, doing the best I knew how to meet the needs of each situation, there seemed to be the sense of inner guidance that I had experienced at other times during the last few years, as well as a sense of support, of strength beyond my own.

There was also a continuing conviction that I should stay with Don. And it truly was where I wanted to be. It was almost as though time stood still, as though I was living in a separate realm with him, apart from the rest of the world. I knew I was getting tired from lack of sleep, but the fatigue didn't seem to affect me adversely. I didn't get sick. I didn't worry about things at home, and was hardly aware of the rest of my life. I was just there . . . there for Don.

On the morning of January 6, Alicia, and another young aide, were talking about trying to lose weight, about the temptation of chocolate. The thought of the box of our favorite chocolates tucked away in Don's dresser drawer popped into my mind. I pulled them out, cut one of the buttercreams in half, and offered it to him.

At first, he was unresponsive. On impulse, I carefully set the piece of candy in his mouth, and slowly his reaction changed. The sweetness seemed to register, and he appeared to be savoring the flavor. I offered him the rest of it, and then a second piece. Although I simply could not interest him in food of any kind, a buttercream seemed to be a different story. I tried a third piece, but his interest had waned.

I wanted to touch base with Sandy and Lisa, but there was no phone in the room — and after the scare with Don's breathing, I was hesitant to leave his side. So that evening when Tom came in to check on him, I asked if he would call and tell them what was going on and how Don was doing. With warmth and caring, he assured me he would be happy to do so.

Late that night Don's roommate, Warren, began saying, "What's the answer?" over and over and over. Finally, half jokingly, and half in frustration, I said, "Warren! What's the question!?" To my dismay, he started repeating both "What's the answer?" and "What's the question?" with "Please help me!" interspersed here and there. Nothing that I said, or tried to do, seemed to help. I was grateful when he finally fell asleep, and the room was quite once again.

A rather confused, but pleasant female resident, who often roamed up and down the halls, wandered in and said, "You're a wonderful woman."

After she shuffled out and on down the hall, I thought about her comment. I didn't feel like a "wonderful woman." There was simply that knowing that I should, and wanted to, be exactly where I was.

I watched with admiration as Ginette and Sharon, two members of the night staff, quietly and patiently moved in and out of each room, doing whatever they could to help the residents settle down for the night.

At 7:00 a.m. the next morning, Becky came in to work with her usual cheerful greeting. Alicia and several other staff members arrived, and could be seen moving up and down the long hall. Again, that sense of awe spread over me. Day after day, the entire staff continued to exhibit the same warmth, sensitivity, and dedication. Their lighthearted humor, which could help the residents over the top of a difficult situation, often brought a smile to my face as well.

Tom appeared in our doorway that afternoon.

"I told the girls you were holding up well, and that you were in charge."

It took a moment for his comment to register. The girls? Then I remembered. I had asked him to call Sandy and Lisa. In charge?

"I am?" My mind was blank. I wasn't sure what he meant.

"Yes. I told them that you are the conductor, and I am only part of the orchestra."

Even then, it took me a while.

Slowly, his meaning began to dawn on me. "Conductor" was not a word I would have chosen. But yes, I was trying to follow my heart, trying to listen for any kind of guidance, and the caring group of people at The Phoenix was compassionately following my lead. The reality, the magnitude of the scene, hit me for a moment. Then almost immediately, my mind jumped back to the challenges of the moment.

Don did not seem to be improving. He still had a temperature, and when the R.N on duty that morning came in to check him, she discovered that his oxygen count was extra low. She asked if I wanted them to use supplementary oxygen.

I thought about her question . . .

Another difficult decision I knew I had to make.

But I knew the answer.

"No . . . thank you," I responded quietly.

Sandy, Lisa, and I each felt strongly that if Don were able to comprehend the present circumstances, and if he were able to tell us his wishes, he would not want us to use measures to try to simply keep him alive. And in each of our minds, it seemed selfish for us to do so.

When the doctor came in a little later, I repeated my request that they not use supplementary oxygen. He looked me in the eye, and with great empathy quietly responded, "I have no problem with that decision."

I was grateful for his similar viewpoint, and thought again how glad I was that Don and I had both filled out living wills and health care proxy forms — and that they both were always there in his charts. I knew that it was essential to have such wishes documented on paper, and also knew that as his health care proxy, it was important for me to be there to back them up.

Tom knew I hated to leave Don's side, but we both knew I needed some sleep. I hurried across the hall to a phone that was on the wall, and called the Fireside to see if "my" room was available. Later that night I talked with Tom, and asked his opinion about leaving for a few hours. What would he do if it were his wife? He checked all of Don's vital signs. For several nights he had said he would probably stay, but tonight, he thought he might go.

I had made a tentative reservation . . .

Late that evening I put my boots on, thinking perhaps I could get up the nerve to move from my spot beside Don's bed and spend a few hours at the motel. He was asleep, and his face looked peaceful and relaxed.

As I thought about the possibility of leaving, I realized the water pitcher was almost out of ice. When I started down the hall to refill it, now wearing my heavy winter boots in place of the slippers, I glanced behind me. Tom was standing by his medication cart in front of the room next to Don's, and happened to look my way.

"I have my boots on," I said with a grin.

"I see," he responded.

From the smile on his face and the twinkle in his eyes, I knew we both understood that short exchange — both knew that I was trying to gather the courage to walk out that night — that I had changed from my slippers to my boots, that I might make it out that door . . .

Sometime around midnight, I did go to the motel — after making sure the number was logged at the desk before I left — and all was well when I walked back into Don's room early the next morning. The owner of the Fireside was always so good about holding the back room for me, if I let him know I might be coming. On one occasion, I made a reservation, but never made it to the motel, and even though he held the room all night, he did not charge me for it.

During those long days and nights, I sometimes played our tapes softly. Sometimes I read to Don. There were times when I simply sat quietly beside him. But often I just talked to him, whether he seemed awake or not. Over the years, we had often joked about how bent his ear was becoming!

I had no idea how much he heard, or whether he could understand my words, but I kept talking.

"I love you so much. You are such a good person — a gentle man, and a gentleman. And amidst all kinds of difficult situations, and in spite of this challenging disease, you have been true to the very special person that you are.

"But now, it really is okay to go. I'll meet you later. Like the laws of cause and effect that we have talked about so often — wherever you are going, I'll come too. I'll meet you there."

Once to my surprise, he mumbled a barely audible, "Okay."

A little later that same evening, he slowly pulled himself up from the bed a little ways, then lay back. He repeated the motion, moving up and back, in what almost looked like a low "situp." His arms were at his sides, but with his eyes, his head and whole upper body, he seemed to be sort of searching or reaching toward something. He appeared to be very preoccupied, as he looked ahead with an intent gaze. He slowly repeated the motion again.

The head of his bed was raised a little bit, but the sight of him raising himself up that far surprised me. He had not been able to sit up by himself since I'd arrived on New Year's Day.

On impulse, I quietly said, "Why don't you lie back and go to sleep?"

"No," he said softly but emphatically.

So I just sat by his side, watching. He did soon relax back onto the bed, but I couldn't help but wonder if I would ever really know what meaning might lie behind what I saw with my eyes. Was he truly hearing my words about something beyond? Could he be glimpsing, and reaching toward, something that he sensed — some reality I could not perceive?

On several occasions I talked to him about the caterpillar-cocoon-butterfly concept that we had discussed many times in the past. It always made such sense to us both. The caterpillar can only crawl along the ground, up trees, and along branches. Then one day it spins a cocoon, and soon appears to be dead. But in time it emerges as a beautiful butterfly that can fly! Perhaps when the human body dies, the spirit is freed, and it, too, is able to "fly," to move on to different dimensions and new horizons.

I spoke about so many things, thinking out loud in the manner I had done so many times over the years.

I read from our books of poetry, and repeated the 23rd Psalm, which had always been a favorite of Don's. I said, and sang, the Lord's Prayer, sang the Irish Blessing, Kumbaya, Eidleweiss, and anything else I could think of.

Sometimes I kissed him gently on the lips. There were times when he did not respond, but once in a while I received the same gentle kiss back.

That heartwarming response always brought tears to my eyes.

The calendar showed January 8, 1995. During the last few days I had often told Don it was "okay to go" — words that came from the depths of my being — words that seemed important to say out loud. Slowly that night, I began to realize that on a few occasions as I sat beside him, thinking about the long, sad road he had walked over the last years, I had quietly said, "Go, Honey . . . "

Suddenly, I was in tears, apologizing — feeling so badly — thinking "Go" was not what I meant to say to this loving husband of mine. My emotions burst forth in a stream of words. "I don't mean to be telling you to go or to stay, Don. You need to do whatever is right for you. I love you so much . . . I don't want to lose you . . . but how can I possibly hold you here? And I do want to be here beside you if you are going to go . . ."

I had been doing fairly well, but at that moment thoughts and feelings of all kinds threatened to overwhelm me. I struggled with my emotions, struggled to keep my balance.

I knew Don Miller. I knew how highly he valued his health, his privacy, his independence, and his freedom. How could I possibly fight to keep him alive under the present circumstances? Yet, how hard to allow him to go, to even encourage him to go — to move on to whatever lay beyond.

What an unbelievable, overwhelming, and unnerving situation.

As I struggled to calm my rattled emotions, I suddenly knew I wanted to talk with David. I needed his perspective, his inputs. I needed to talk with him in person — to think "out loud" about the thoughts and feelings that threatened to erode my composure.

I moved across the hall to use the phone, reached David's answering machine and left a message. He soon called back. Would he have time to see me tomorrow afternoon? He would make time, was his quiet response. We agreed on four o'clock.

I also needed to go home to get some different clothes. It would take me an hour to get there, 45 minutes to get to David's office, and another hour to get back to The Phoenix. I would have to be gone most of the afternoon and early evening. "Do I dare be away from Don for that length of time?" I asked myself.

I hesitatingly approached Becky and Alicia. Would they mind sitting with Don while I was gone so that he wouldn't be alone?

They both readily agreed. Taking turns, I discovered later, they used personal time to do so. What special young women they were. Great kindness and understanding could be seen in their eyes, and reflected through their gentle responses.

I hurried home, thankful that the roads were dry on that cold January day. I rushed through my closet and drawers to find the things I needed, then hurried to David's office, and back to The Phoenix. I breathed a sigh of relief and gratefulness, as I settled back in our chair next to Don's bed that evening — relief that I had made the round trip with no mishap, grateful for Becky and Alicia, grateful for David's support and listening ear, and most of all, grateful that Don's condition had not worsened while I was gone.

As I sat next to him that evening, I suddenly realized that he seemed a little more alert. His eyes were open and appeared to be more focused. An idea began to form in my mind. Sandy and Lisa — could I call them? Perhaps let him hear their voices? Could we possibly get him down to the desk, where there was a phone he could reach? I knew he could not sit or stand alone — knew that such an undertaking would be a huge challenge.

As I sat there wondering, Lee, another of the special members of that caring staff, walked into Don's room. I asked what she thought about my idea, and was delighted with her ready willingness to see if we could manage it. She went off to find a wheelchair. We struggled to get Don into it, shared a look of triumph when we succeeded, and were soon on our way down the hall to the desk.

I dialed Lisa's number, and after several rings, was very glad to hear her familiar voice respond. We talked for a few moments. I explained the situation, then put the receiver to Don's ear.

What an awesome thing it was to watch the look on his face, as her voice appeared to, somehow, slowly register. I knew she would be reminding him of some special times they had together, telling him that he was a wonderful dad, telling him how much she loved him. He grinned, laughed, even tried to respond to her! After we hung up, he seemed excited — almost "punch drunk." What an unbelievable change it was from the unresponsiveness of previous days. I had wondered, had hoped, but had no real idea if such a call to our daughter could register in his mind. I was well aware that he probably was not able to retain the memory of those moments, but they were unforgettable ones for me to observe.

It wasn't until later, that I learned how difficult it had been for Lisa after she hung up that phone . . . What a special gift her voice was. I will always be grateful for her efforts, for her sincere and loving response that evening.

I tried Sandy's number, was disappointed to be greeted by their answering machine, then suddenly remembered what day it was. It was tomorrow that she planned to fly up from North Carolina. I was sorry not to reach her on that special night, but so glad that she was planning to come.

Lee reappeared. We wheeled Don back to his room, and she helped me get him into bed. He was soon asleep. As I watched his relaxed face that held just the hint of a grin, I was thankful for those few brief moments in time, for that bit of clarity, for the love that flowed from Lisa to Don through that telephone receiver.

On the evening of January 10, Sandy arrived at our airport with Katie and Christy for a two-day visit. She rented a car, stayed at the house, and drove over to Vermont the next morning. Many of the residents were sick, and I was hesitant to have her bring three-month-old Christy into the nursing home. But it was important to Sandy to have both girls come in, and soon all four of us were gathered around Don's bed in that little room.

Sandy had carefully talked in advance with "almost" four-year-old Katie.

"Grandad's eyes may be closed. He may look like he's asleep, like he's not listening. But just pretend that he's listening. His ears work. He can hear anything you say, and don't worry if he doesn't talk back to you."

How heartwarming it was to watch Katie. She stood beside the bed for a moment looking at Don. Then she reached up and patted her grandad's arm, stretched up on her tiptoes to give him a kiss, and said in her sincere little voice, "I love you, Grandad."

We saw no visible response from Don, but when Sandy and I looked at one another, we both knew we had responded to Katie, as we struggled to maintain our composure.

Katie was soon busily coloring in her new coloring book, while Sandy and I talked quietly, consciously including Don in our conversation, even though he could not actually participate. His eyes were closed, but Sandy's words to Katie had come from the bottom of her heart. Even though we saw no outward signs to prove it, we both firmly believed that he might be able to sense our presence, hear our words.

When the three of them came back the next day, I took Katie and Christy over to the Fireside for a few hours. The moments of alertness that had suddenly appeared two days earlier seemed to have passed, but both Sandy and I knew it was important for her to have some time alone with her dad.

When they left our house in New York early the following day, two special friends of ours helped Sandy and the girls get to the nearby airport. Katie and Christy were in our friends' car while Sandy drove the rental car. As they pulled away from the house, Katie, who had never met these two adults before and was now with them in a strange car, said, "I miss my mom . . . " When Christy made a few singing noises, Katie mustered up her courage and said, "It's okay, Christy, I'm here."

Yes, Katie, I understood. You were a little afraid. You thought Christy might be too, and you wanted to reassure her, wanted to let her know that you were there for her.

I, too, am a little afraid. I think your grandad might be too . . . and I want to reassure him, want to let him know I am here for him.

That evening, after Sandy, Katie, and Christy left, I was singing to Don. "Bell-bottom trousers, coat of navy blue, she loves a sailor, and he loves her, too," was softly rolling out when

I realized that it was a Navy song. Don was in the Air Force for two years, not the Navy! This was not the proper song to be singing! I sat there thinking and thinking, but simply could not remember the Air Force anthem. I knew Warren was awake. Could he remember? Would he respond?

I called over to him quietly, "Hey, Warren, what's the Air Force song?" Silence. Then all of a sudden, from behind the curtain around the next bed came, "Off we go, into the wild blue yonder . . ." Then he suddenly stopped.

"That's great! What comes next, Warren?" I could not seem to remember.

Even now, I'm not exactly sure what he came up with, but it seemed right. I think it was, "Climbing high, into the sky." Whatever his contribution was, we sang those words together, along with some others we came up with, quietly blending our not-so-mellow voices in the small room of that nursing home.

A little later that night, I was just sitting in the quiet room, watching Don. On impulse, I leaned over and gave him a big, long, full kiss.

And . . . he returned it! With great intensity!

I had not expected much of a response, burst into tears, and struggled with my efforts to say, "Thank you, Honey!"

How many years had it been since he had kissed me full on the mouth . . . in such a meaningful way . . . I simply could not remember how long it had been.

Even if that "kiss" might have been some kind of automatic response to mine, the fact that I knew it was how he would respond if he possibly could, made it an incredible . . . unforgettable . . . moment in time.

Chapter Fourteen

Don continued to have no interest in food, but he would still take ice quite readily, and occasionally sips of water. I was beginning to lose track of time, but one day when I went to get ice for him, I noticed the calendar at the nurse's station. January 14. It had been two weeks since I had arrived at The Phoenix on the first day of 1995.

That morning, the doctor came in to check Don, and told me that his left lung was almost blocked, that the right one was very raspy. A little later, the aides and I noticed that for the first time Don flinched, obviously in pain when we moved him.

Around 8:00 that evening, the doctor was back to examine him again.

"Both lungs seem better," he said quietly. "Things could go either way.

"I saw the notation in Don's chart about pain," he added, "and I have prescribed morphine. It is there, if he needs it."

Don slept much of the evening. Ginette and Sharon came in together to check on him, and to change him. All three of us watched his face as they worked. He began to wince . . . causing each of us to wince as well.

We looked at one another.

We couldn't let Don hurt.

Ginette quietly left, and returned with the morphine that the doctor had made sure was available.

Don's body felt cold to our touch. She brought in another blanket.

Late into that night I sat next to Don, watching. He began to seem more comfortable and relaxed, but his hand and arm felt cold — even though they were underneath both blankets.

Perhaps my body could help keep his warm.

He lay on his back, as he always seemed to do in the nursing home. I gently lay down beside him "upside down" on the bed. I carefully slipped my feet under his pillow, and placed a small pillow from home by his feet for my head.

From that vantage point, I could see that his feet were not fully covered. They felt so cold. I gently massaged them, then carefully pulled the blankets over them.

I was almost asleep, when Sharon came in to check on Don. "Enjoy the closeness," she said quietly.

Her smile was warm, kind, and understanding, but I suddenly realized how strange the scene might appear to others! How I appreciated the caring tone, the complete acceptance of my constant presence, and now, of my position on that narrow hospital bed.

I awoke a little later, and cautiously slipped off the bed. Don appeared to be comfortable, and was sleeping peacefully.

I checked my watch. It was 3:00 a.m. I realized how very tired I was . . . and asked myself a familiar question. "Do I dare leave?"

A few hours sleep on a motel bed sounded so appealing . . .

Earlier that night, I had asked the Fireside owners to reserve "my" room . . . just in case . . .

I tucked the blankets around Don, gave him a kiss, and tiptoed out, down the hall, and by the desk, determined to give it a try.

"I'm going to the Fireside," I told Ginette, and then Sharon, when I met her as she came out of one of the rooms near the door of the unit. "Please watch carefully, and call me if you see any change."

They both assured me they would.

I didn't even take my clothes off when I got to the motel room. I just stretched out on that bed and was sound asleep almost immediately. At 7:00 a.m., I was suddenly wide awake. No one had called, but I knew I needed to get back to Don. In a matter of minutes, I drove the few blocks between the motel and The Phoenix, arrived back in Don's room, and settled into the chair beside his bed.

The R.N. on duty that morning popped in for a moment. "Don appeared to be in pain at 5:00 a.m., so they gave him morphine. He seems comfortable now, but we will watch, and use it whenever we think he needs it," she reported.

My "Thanks so much," came from the bottom of my heart. I hadn't been there, Ginette and Sharon knew it, and they did watch carefully. I was deeply grateful.

Don did seem very relaxed, and was breathing easily. But when his eyes were open, they were often staring — with such a vacant look . . .

A little later that morning, Becky appeared at the door of Don's room. "Mike called," she told me. "He said to tell you that he is planning to drive over tonight, and will do so unless he hears from you."

I thanked her, then glanced out the window on that cold winter morning. It would be a long, windy, and snowy drive for Mike. Did he have some sense that a visit was important on that particular night? How many, many times Mike had been there for us, turned up when we needed him most, always with a cheerful grin, and a caring hug.

Don seemed to be asleep, as the two of us sat next to his bed and talked quietly that evening. I was grateful for Mike's company, grateful for the special effort he had made to be there.

Our little corner of that nursing home seemed so still after Mike left. Warren was asleep on the other side of the curtain. I set the volume level very low and slipped our *My Fair Lady* tape into the cassette player, then the *Strauss Waltz* tape. As the mellow strains of the familiar music drifted along, Don opened his eyes, and appeared to be aware of my presence. I gently kissed him all over his face, in a joking kind of manner . . . and just the hint of a smile appeared.

Before long, he slipped back to sleep. His arms were on top of the covers, and I suddenly realized they felt cold — almost clammy. They looked sort of mottled and a bit bluish, as his skin had for a number of days. I massaged them a little, trying to warm them, then carefully tucked and retucked the blankets around him.

I studied that familiar face for a long time. He looked so relaxed. I noticed that a small reddish blue spot had appeared on the top of his left ear.

I sat quietly, watching Don Miller . . . as he lay there, so still . . .

Lee came in to check on him, and we tried to assess the situation. He continued to seem comfortable when he was still, but in spite of the morphine, it obviously caused him pain when we tried to gently move him to change the diapers. A silent look between us was all we needed. We would not use them. Causing any further pain for Don was something neither one of us wanted to do.

We worked together at gently moving him, and slipped a pad under, and a towel over him. His arms and legs were so thin . . .

I was so tired, but somehow knew I should not leave again. I moved the chair very close to the bed. I stroked Don's arm, ran my hand across his hair and onto his neck. I watched him . . . and talked to him quietly.

About 1:00 a.m, his breathing seemed to change. Something was . . . different . . .

Ginette was on duty, and I called to her softly, as she silently moved past our door on her way down the quiet hall. She came in quickly. She checked Don's vital signs, looked at me, shook her head slightly, and remained with us, her fingers gently touching the pulse on his wrist.

She stood on the other side of the bed, and as the two of us watched, Don's breaths slowly became sort of gasps, almost as though he had come in from a long run.

I had been talking to him when she walked in, and had paused. With obvious compassion, Ginette whispered, "Keep talking . . ."

Struggling to maintain my composure, I quietly repeated the words that had rolled out so often over the last two weeks. "It's okay to go, Don. If you see a Light, sense a Love, it's all right to follow it. Like when you left for Tokyo with the Air Force, and I couldn't go with you, but came later, I will come later again this time . . . I will meet you. Wait for me, and don't go too far away . . . I love you so very much. I know you love me, but it's okay to go . . . okay to go . . . okay to go . . . "

Gradually the pauses between his breaths became longer and longer . . .

Then . . . his breathing simply stopped.

It was 1:30 a.m.

Ginette asked if I was all right, then quietly slipped out of the room.

For a while, I just sat . . . sat there next to Don . . .

Then I stood up . . . stood beside him, looking at the face I knew so well . . . Finally, I leaned over and kissed him on the cheek, then walked to the door and down the hall toward the desk.

I called the funeral home where I had made advance arrangements. The best thing to do at that hour of the night was to call someone there in Vermont, said the female voice on the other end of the line. She would do that right away.

I went back to Don's room, sat down, and one last time, gently moved my hand across his hair and slipped it down the side of his neck. It was warm, but the rest of him was rapidly becoming colder. Already his face was gray.

He was so still.

But . . . it was only a body that lay on that bed.

I really knew that Don was not there.

This body was only his "space suit" — for use in this material world of ours. He didn't need it anymore. The idea had always made such sense to me . . . and at that moment, there was no doubt in my mind.

Yet . . . I continued to struggle with my thoughts and emotions.

"How does one cope with watching a loved one slip away!?" I wondered.

The people from the funeral home arrived . . . I moved down to the desk. They took Don's body out on a gurney . . . in a body bag.

In so many ways, it all seemed completely unreal.

In spite of the hour, and per their requests, I called Sandy and Lisa.

I hesitatingly dialed the number Becky had given me. She too had said, "Please call . . . "

Then I called the Fireside, and the sleepy voice of the owner finally responded. "I'm sorry about your husband," he said, "Of course I'll leave a key in the box for you."

Finally, there was nothing more I could do. Functioning on some kind of automatic pilot, I walked down that hall, out the door to the car, and headed for the motel. As I drove down the familiar street in the middle of that unforgettable night, it dawned on me.

The funeral home that had been called was directly across the street from the Fireside Motel. Don's body would be there that night, right across the street from where I would be.

I knew they would take it to the hospital at home the next day . . . to remove his brain for an autopsy and research. I knew they would then take it to the crematorium.

I wondered again. How on earth does one deal with such a scene . . .

But I was discovering the answer to that question.

Somehow, one just does . . . by putting one foot in front of the other . . . by taking that one step . . . that one moment at a time.

At first, I simply felt numb as I took off my well-worn jeans and sweatshirt, pulled on my nightgown, and stretched out on the bed in that motel room. My mind was blank. I could hardly believe all that had just happened.

Slowly my thoughts moved back in time . . . replayed those almost incomprehensible moments . . .

How grateful I was that I had shared so many thoughts with Don . . . that I had told him how much I loved him. I had read many times that hearing was the last thing to go . . . I didn't know if he had truly been able to "hear". . . but I had said the words . . . and some part of me knew that some part of him had understood.

And how very grateful I was to have been with him those last 16 days . . . and there when he left.

As I lay in the stillness, I knew something else.

It was right not to treat anything . . . right to let him go. He was free.

I didn't know so long ago when I was looking for my "special someone," that one could love so deeply that it would be possible to let that someone go — let that someone die.

In spite of the fatigue, and amidst the deep sadness that enveloped me, a sense of peace, of all-rightness began to drift into my heart. A sense that would surely come and go, but for that moment, I breathed a sigh of thankfulness, a sigh of relinquishment.

And I slept.